What to Expect When You Have Diabetes

What to Expect When You Have Diabetes

Diabetes

 Tips for
Living Well with Diabetes

Revised & Updated

by the

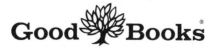

Foreword by John Buse, MD, PHD

Good 🌳 Books®

New York, New York

Copyright © 2016 by Good Books, an imprint of Skyhorse Publishing, Inc.

All rights reserved. No part of this book may be reproduced in any manner without the express written consent of the publisher, except in the case of brief excerpts in critical reviews or articles. All inquiries should be addressed to Good Books, 307 West 36th Street, 11th Floor, New York, NY 10018.

Good Books is an imprint of Skyhorse Publishing, Inc.®, a Delaware corporation. Visit our website at www.goodbooks.com.

10 9 8 7 6 5 4 3 2 1

Library of Congress Cataloging-in-Publication data is available on file

Print ISBN: 978-1-68099-144-4
ebook ISBN: 978-1-68099-145-1

Printed in the United States of America

TABLE OF CONTENTS

Sugar

Fat

Dining Out

General

FOREWORD

We are in the midst of a world-wide epidemic. According to the World Health Organization, in 2014, about 347 million people had diabetes (world-wide). In 2015, there were about 415 million adults with diabetes. The epidemic is increasing at an alarming rate. Whether you have diabetes yourself or whether you are a caregiver to someone who does, this book will help you understand what diabetes is and how to cope with its many challenges. Written in a clear, easy-to-read question-and-answer format, this book puts a wealth of diabetes information at your fingertips.

Diabetes is a chronic disease that affects how a person produces and responds to insulin. Insulin is the hormone key that unlocks your body's cells, allowing sugars to enter and provide energy. If cells become resistant to insulin or if we don't make enough insulin, our bodies simply will not work properly. People with type 2 diabetes typically have no symptoms unless their blood sugar level is at least twice normal, and then the symptoms can be fairly subtle and common even in people without diabetes—fatigue, irritability, getting up at night to urinate. If left unchecked, elevated blood sugar can cause peripheral artery disease, nerve damage in legs and feet, degenerating eyesight, kidney failure, and heart disease. Therefore, diabetes is a disease that has to be sought out and treated to avoid complications. Waiting for symptoms can be too late to prevent disability.

There are several main types of diabetes. Type 1 occurs when the body attacks and destroys the cells in the pancreas that produce insulin. Generally affecting young people, type 1 diabetes requires a person to inject insulin daily in order to control his or her blood-sugar levels.

Type 2 diabetes develops more gradually and, while it typically affects people later in life, it is increasingly common in younger people. It is the most common form of the disease. It starts when the body becomes more resistant to insulin, reducing its ability to regulate blood sugar. Over time, this leads to an increase in blood-sugar levels that, if ignored, can lead to major health problems.

This book is weighted heavily toward people with type 2 diabetes, primarily because 95% of the people who have diabetes have this type. Type 1 is much more rare, but except for a few instances, most of the treatment and lifestyle suggestions are helpful for both.

Gestational diabetes is another type that affects between about 4 and 9% of all pregnant women. Gestational diabetes tends to go away after the pregnancy, but it can increase your risk of getting diabetes later in life.

If you have diabetes, what should you do? Awareness is the best defense, and offense. Talk to your doctor, nurse, and diabetes educator. They will help you learn more about how to control your blood glucose, blood pressure, and blood lipids, and teach you preventive care for your eyes, kidneys, and feet by maintaining a healthier lifestyle through proper diet and increased activity.

And finally, if there's one message I would like to give to all the readers of this book, it is "Take care of yourself." Learn as much as you can about diabetes. Know why you feel the way you do and what to expect. Learn how to recognize changes. Try new recipes. Walk more. Live life to its fullest by making healthy choices. And don't be shy about asking questions and being an active partner in your health-care team. It's your diabetes and your life. And the ADA is here to help you.

John Buse, MD, PhD
(President, Medicine & Science, American Diabetes Association)

Now That You Have Diabetes

1 Is diabetes a new disease?

No. Diabetes was identified 2,000 years ago by Aretaeus of Cappadocia, the Greek physician. However, very little progress was made in understanding or treating the disease until 1869 when Paul Langerhans described small islands (islets) in the pancreas. However, he did not know their function in regulating blood-sugar levels. In 1889, German scientist Oskar Minkowski discovered a critical link between the pancreas and diabetes when he removed a dog's pancreas and observed that it caused the dog to urinate frequently. He also found sugar in the dog's urine.

In 1909, the Belgian scientist Jean de Meyer used the term "insulin" to describe a hypothetical substance in the pancreas that controls blood sugar, even though insulin had not yet been discovered. Finally in 1921, after a series of experiments, J.J.R. Macleod,

Charles Best, Frederick Banting, and James Collip succeeded in purifying insulin and successfully treating a diabetes patient with it. This discovery saved many people from dying in a coma due to high blood sugars. Although diabetes has been around a long time, we still need new and better therapies.

2 What does the term "diabetes mellitus" mean?

"Diabetes" and "mellitus" have two different histories and meanings. "Diabetes" is usually attributed to the Greek physician Aretaeus, who lived in 200 BC. He used the term "diabetes," meaning "to siphon or to flow through," for a disease in which the water that a person drinks runs rapidly through his or her body. It was not until the end of the 18th century that the term "mellitus" was added to "diabetes." An Englishman, John Rollo, and a German, Johann Peter Frank, first used the term "mellitus" (which means "sweet as honey") in the medical literature to describe the sweetness of the urine. So "diabetes mellitus" literally means a medical condition in which the patient drinks too much water and urinates frequently. The urine is sweet because it contains sugar.

3 Can I catch diabetes from someone else?

No. Diabetes is not like a cold or the flu. You cannot catch it from other people, even by kissing them. There are many causes of diabetes, but no form of diabetes has ever been shown to be infectious or contagious. Most diabetes develops from an inherited tendency to get it. If you have inherited this gene, you may develop type 1 diabetes when you are exposed to something in the environment. This unknown factor triggers the onset of diabetes. You may develop type 2 diabetes if (in addition to the gene) you gain weight and don't exercise regularly. There are also less common causes of diabetes, such as prolonged, excessive drinking of alcohol or having too much iron in your blood. So while there are many causes of diabetes, catching it from another person is not one of them.

4 Is there a time of year when I am more likely to get diabetes?

Yes and no. Many studies have been done to determine when people get diabetes. Type 1 diabetes (previously called "insulin-dependent diabetes") usually occurs in thin individuals less than 30 years of age. It is more common to develop type 1 diabetes in the fall, the season in which many viral infections occur (for example, chicken pox, influenza, and the measles). Some experts think the higher rate of type 1 diabetes during the fall months suggests that type 1 diabetes may be started by a virus that causes an infection. However, this has never been proven. Type 2 diabetes generally appears gradually and has never been linked to a specific time of year.

5 Does eating sugar cause diabetes?

No. Although diabetes has been called "sugar diabetes" for many years, eating sugar does not cause it.
Type 1 diabetes happens when your body's immune
system destroys the insulin-producing beta-cells in the
pancreas. Factors that may cause the immune system
to do this are autoantibodies, cow's milk, genetics,
and oxygen-free radicals. Type 1 diabetes is probably
triggered by one of these environmental factors in
people who have the genes for developing the disease.
Type 2 diabetes is often the result of a combination
of factors, including genetics and lifestyle. However,
eating sugar, while possibly contributing to weight
gain, is not a cause.

6 Is diabetes a dangerous disease?

Yes. Statistics prove that diabetes causes much suffering and lost work time. It is the leading cause of kidney failure and the seventh leading cause of death in this country. Each year in the United States, between 15,000 and 30,000 people lose their eyesight because of diabetes, and 160,000 individuals die from diabetes-related causes. In fact, during the last 20 years, diabetes has caused more deaths than have all of the wars throughout the world in the 20th century. Unfortunately, the situation is getting worse, not better: the number of people developing diabetes is increasing. We all need to do our best to prevent and treat this disease in the United States and throughout the world.

7 Can I ignore the risks of diabetic complications since the thought of them scares me?

No, because taking action now can prevent the disabling complications of diabetes. Adjusting your food, physical activity, and medication (if any) to bring your blood-sugar levels to near normal ranges can help you avoid or delay complications. Research has proven that.

It's very common for people to fear aging or becoming disabled, whether or not they have diabetes. We all want to live well every day that we have, and be fully functional and independent. But choosing to ignore the effects of diabetes won't make them go away. Rather, taking charge to change the outcome can give you peace of mind, so you can live your life without fear. Knowing the effects of diabetic complications on your body is information that can give you power over the future!

8 How close are we to a cure for diabetes?

It depends on what you mean by a cure. Diabetes is not really one disease. It has many causes and, therefore, many cures. Recent years saw significant advances in diabetes prevention and treatment. These advances are important until cures become available. The ultimate cure for diabetes will likely involve replacing the cells in the pancreas that make insulin. Blood sugars can be more easily controlled by inserting a remote-controlled insulin pump that is automatically regulated by a glucose sensor. The implantable pump has already been developed and tested in more than 400 people worldwide. Glucose sensors are under development and should be available soon.

9 How do I know whether I have type 1, type 2, or another type of diabetes?

With type 1 diabetes, the body stops making insulin, often before, during, or shortly after adolescence (though there is no cut-off age). People with type 1 diabetes require insulin for life because insulin is essential for using and storing food. These people are usually lean and, without insulin, would go into a diabetic coma within a day or two. In the past, this disease was called "insulin-dependent diabetes mellitus" (IDDM). The proper name is now type 1 diabetes.

People with type 2 diabetes have enough insulin early in the disease, but their bodies are unable to use the insulin correctly to lower blood sugar. They are insulin resistant. Most people with type 2 diabetes are overweight and more than 30 years old when diagnosed. Often, people with type 2 diabetes can control their blood sugar with diet and exercise, though some take oral diabetes pills. After several years with type 2 diabetes, many people eventually need insulin as the disease progresses. In the past, this type of diabetes was called "non-insulin-dependent diabetes mellitus" (NIDDM). The correct term is now type 2 diabetes.

10 Should I tell my boss and coworkers that I have diabetes?

Whether or not to tell anyone is up to you. Your coworkers are not responsible for taking care of you, but you will probably find that they will be understanding and want to help you stay healthy. You do have a responsibility to yourself and your coworkers to keep the work environment safe. It is important to have a system in place for managing emergencies, such as severely low blood sugar or a sick day. Most people feel more comfortable dealing with emergencies when they have some preparation and understanding. You don't have to make diabetes the daily topic of conversation, and you may feel uncomfortable letting people at work become the "control patrol." This is a personal choice that requires consideration on your part, but you may find that your life is easier if you allow others to support you in managing your diabetes and staying healthy.

11 What is a health-care team and how can I find one?

In addition to your primary care provider (doctor, nurse practitioner, or physician assistant), you need someone trained to help you with the day-to-day challenges of living with diabetes. A certified diabetes educator (CDE) is a health professional who has been trained and certified as an expert in diabetes education and management. The CDE may be a registered nurse (RN), registered dietician (RD), pharmacist, or another physician.

You can locate a CDE in your area online at www. diabeteseducator.org, or by calling the American Association of Diabetes Educators (AADE) Awareness Hotline at (800) TEAM-UP4. They will ask for your zip code and help you find a CDE near you. If you cannot find a CDE, you may find a nurse or RD who is interested in diabetes and willing to help you. Your doctor may also refer you to someone with experience in diabetes care.

You may also want to find a diabetes education program that offers individual or group classes. The ADA has a list of recognized diabetes programs in your area. Call (800) DIABETES for this information. If there isn't a recognized diabetes center near you, call your local hospital and ask about a diabetes education program or about diabetes educators on staff.

12 How often should I see my doctor to be as healthy as I can be?

The frequency of medical visits required to manage your diabetes varies according to numerous factors: (1) how long you've had diabetes, (2) your ability to adjust your treatment regimen effectively to maintain good blood-sugar control, and (3) whether you have diabetic complications or other medical problems that may interfere with your diabetes management.

At a minimum, all patients with diabetes should see a doctor twice a year. Recharging your motivation to achieve good blood-sugar control is an important part of every visit. You should also have an A1C test (see Glossary) at each semi-annual visit to test your average blood-sugar levels over a period of two or three months. Or if you are on insulin, you should take the test quarterly to monitor your blood-sugar control.

In addition, every patient with diabetes should have someone he or she can contact on short notice to discuss problems as they arise, such as unexplained high blood sugars or sudden illness. This person need not be a physician but may be a certified diabetes educator (CDE), registered dietitian (RD), nurse practitioner, or nurse case manager.

13   Is there a list of tests and things I am supposed to do to stay healthy?

Yes. The ADA publishes "Standards of Medical Care for Patients with Diabetes Mellitus" to provide guidelines for health professionals to manage diabetes and prevent complications. We recommend a checklist based on those standards to help diabetes patients keep track of all that needs to be done (see below and on page 33). Some tests come every three months and others yearly. For instance, you should have your eyes checked by an ophthalmologist and your urine checked for microalbuminuria (small amounts of protein) yearly. With these two tests, your doctor can detect eye and kidney problems early and start treatment. You may want to use your own flow sheet to be sure you get the tests done at the right time and to share these results with your health-care team. Talk with your team about which of these tests you need and when you should have each one done.

Self-Care Checklist

Self-Care Activities	Frequency	Date(s) to be Completed
Review blood-sugar log. (A1C Goal _____)	*Quarterly*	
Review blood-pressure log.	*Quarterly*	
Ophthalmology: Dilated exam to check for glaucoma and cataracts.	*Annually*	
Flu Vaccinations (Pneumovax)	*Annually*	

Self-Care Activities	Frequency	Date(s) to be Completed
Kidney: Albuminuria screen BUN/Creatinine	*Annually*	
Neuropathy/Feet: Get a comprehensive foot exam. *(Check feet and legs daily for sores, corns, calluses, and cuts.)*	*Annually*	
Cardiovascular: Check blood pressure and get a baseline EKG. Lipids screening (fasting).	*Quarterly* *At initial medical evaluation, and periodically after that*	
Hypoglycemia/ Hyperglycemia: Review management plan. If it is prescribed, have Glucagon on hand.	*Monthly*	
Diabetes Education	*Initial review at diagnosis, and annually after that*	
Hospitalizations (List reasons)		

14 How can I tell if my diabetes program is successful?

Keep track of your diabetes the same way you do your checking account—by keeping tabs on the balance. With diabetes, the balance is the sum of:

- Your blood sugar
- Your daily weight
- Your blood pressure
- Your level of exercise
- How you feel

If all of these items meet your goals, then you are doing fine.

Keep a daily record of your blood sugar and weight. You can check your blood pressure at home or have it done at shopping centers or pharmacies. Make daily exercise one of your goals. When you monitor your health daily, you help yourself succeed.

Example of a Daily Self-Care Record

Date	Weight	Blood Pressure	Average Glucose	Feelings	Exercise
6/1	150	122/80	102	Good	Yes
6/2	151	120/75	111	Good	No
6/3	149	115/80	98	So/So	Yes

BLOOD-SUGAR HIGHS AND LOWS

15 What are the symptoms of high blood sugar?

The symptoms of high blood sugar may vary from person to person or even in one person from day to day. But, in general, a person will:

1. Feel more hungry or thirsty than usual
2. Have to urinate more frequently than normal
3. Have to get up at night several times to go to the bathroom
4. Feel very tired or sleepy or have no energy
5. Be unable to see clearly or see "halos" when looking at a light

If you have any of these symptoms, check your glucose immediately. Do not treat these symptoms with additional insulin unless you are certain that they are due to high blood sugar. There are other conditions that cause similar symptoms.

16 What type of damage does high blood sugar do to my body?

Over time, high blood-sugar levels can damage both blood vessels and nerves in your body. This can result in poor blood flow to your hands, feet, legs, arms, and vital organs. Poor blood flow to these areas increases your risk of infections, heart problems, stroke, blindness, foot or leg amputation, and kidney disease. In addition, you can lose feeling in your feet or have increased pain in your feet and legs. Even mild injuries can damage your feet without your knowing it. Finally, damage to blood vessels and nerves can lead to sexual problems that are difficult to treat. For all these reasons, you should make a major effort to avoid high blood sugars in your body.

17 What are my blood-sugar goals if I have diabetes?

Try for nearly normal blood-sugar levels with few episodes of low blood sugar. The ADA's goals are shown in the chart below. They are determined from studies that examined the effects of near normal blood-sugar levels on the rates of diabetic complications. If you are persistently outside of these goals or have low blood sugar too often, discuss changing your diabetes therapy with your health-care team.

Target Blood-Sugar Levels for People with Diabetes (mg/dl)

	Nondiabetic Levels	Goal Levels	Action Needed
Before-meal blood sugar	<100	70–130	<70 or >200
After-meal blood sugar	<180 at 1-2 hours after eating	180	<100 or >180
A1C (hemoglobin levels)	<6%	<7% (Individualize with the help of your diabetes specialist)	8%

< means "less than"   > means "greater than"

18 Should I be concerned about glucose control if I have type 2 diabetes?

Yes, but maybe not "tight" control. The older you were when you developed diabetes, the less benefit you get from achieving excellent glucose control. Because the benefits of tight control can differ depending on your age and situation, you and your health-care team need to determine your risk before you decide what your target A1C should be. (For more on A1C, see Glossary and chart on page 37 for target A1C levels.)

The Veterans Health Administration (VHA) has developed guidelines specific to the age at which you developed type 2 diabetes. These guidelines are now used in all Veterans Affairs (VA) clinics. For example, a patient who developed type 2 diabetes at an elderly age may have a target A1C of about 9%, whereas younger patients may benefit from a lower A1C of 7%. For details on these guidelines and what your target A1C should be, ask your health provider for information on this subject.

19 Why should I work so hard to improve my blood-sugar level?

You'll feel more energy and a greater sense of well-being when your blood sugar enters the normal range. In addition, you'll delay or prevent problems with your eyes, kidneys, and nerves as your blood sugar improves. Many doctors also believe that problems with heart disease, stroke, and hardening of the arteries may be delayed by good blood-sugar control. If you do not get these complications of diabetes, you'll live a longer, healthier life.

20 Should I take vitamins or minerals to improve my blood sugar?

There is not enough scientific evidence to recommend vitamin or mineral supplements to improve your blood sugar. From time to time, various vitamin and mineral supplements have been popular. Magnesium, chromium, zinc, vanadium, and selenium have been promoted by health-food stores as having a beneficial effect on blood sugar. However, eating foods that contain the vitamins and minerals, such as fruits and vegetables, is still the best way to get what your body needs.

In addition, we strongly recommend that you get pneumonia vaccinations (available all year) and annual flu vaccinations (available in early fall). Vaccinations may prevent, or reduce the severity of, these illnesses, which usually cause high blood sugars. See page 32 for additional vaccination advice. Ask your health-care team for advice.

21   How will alcohol affect my blood sugar?

Alcohol interferes with your body's ability to produce blood sugar, resulting in low blood sugar. Do not drink alcohol if you are not eating. If you are eating a meal and you drink only a small quantity of alcohol, then the alcohol should not cause low blood sugar. Women should not consume more than one serving of alcohol per day, and men should not consumer more than two. You will need to include the calories that are in the alcohol in your meal plan. In general, one alcoholic beverage equals one alcohol equivalent in a meal plan. Check with your registered dietitian (RD) for help with this. (The ADA provides exchange lists for nearly 700 foods. Search online for *Choose Your Foods: Exchanges Lists for Diabetes.*)

22 How does being overweight affect my ability to obtain normal blood sugars?

Being overweight causes resistance to insulin. This means that any insulin your body makes (or that you inject) will have a hard time lowering your blood sugar. This makes good blood-sugar control difficult. In addition, being overweight may raise your blood pressure, which makes you prone to kidney disease and stroke. Often high blood-fat levels, which contribute to heart disease, also are associated with being overweight. All things considered, reducing your weight will improve your blood-sugar levels and your health.

23 Will I gain weight as I lower my blood sugar?

Not necessarily, especially if you keep track of how much you eat. However, many people do gain weight, and the reasons are complex. One factor is that you are no longer losing large quantities of calories in your urine in the form of glucose. You will need to eliminate calories from your diet equal to what was being lost in your urine. You won't know how many calories this is unless you closely monitor your weight and what you eat. If you start to gain weight, reduce the amount of food you eat and exercise more. If lowering your blood sugar causes you to have more low blood-sugar reactions, then the food that you eat to treat the reactions may add to weight gain.

24 How does the health of my teeth affect my blood sugar?

People with diabetes often have chronic gum disease, which may affect blood-sugar levels. You should make an appointment with a dentist for a comprehensive gum examination and have your teeth professionally cleaned at least twice a year because gum disease is more severe in people with diabetes than people without diabetes.

Gum disease results from the formation of plaque underneath the gum line after eating. Plaque hardens into tartar, which irritates the gums and gradually erodes the underlying bone that holds the teeth in place. Thus, gum disease can lead to the need for dentures. Daily dental care can prevent gum disease from starting. Brush your teeth at least twice a day with a soft-bristle brush and floss daily. Flossing removes food from between the teeth, and plaque from the gum line.

25 How often should I see my doctor to keep my blood sugar under control?

Upon an initial diagnosis, you will need to see your doctor weekly or every two weeks. How often you see your doctor, registered dietitian (RD), or diabetes educator will depend on how long you have had diabetes, your ability to adjust your medication for tight blood-sugar control, and whether you have any diabetic complications or other medical problems that may interfere with your diabetes management. After that, a visit every three months may be enough to reach your target goals.

At a minimum, you should plan on seeing your doctor twice a year to arrange for necessary eye and kidney checkups and to stay motivated about good blood-sugar control. You should have someone you can contact on short notice to discuss problems as they arise, such as unexplained high blood sugars or sudden illness. This person does not have to be a physician but may be a certified diabetes educator (CDE), RD, nurse practitioner, or nurse case manager.

26 Where can I find new information that will help me with my blood-sugar management?

There are several ways to find out about new discoveries and products that will help you control your blood-sugar levels. You can call the ADA's home office at 800 DIABETES, or call 888 DIABETES to find the ADA office nearest you. They may have information about new products and techniques to treat diabetes. You can subscribe to *Diabetes Forecast*, a magazine for people with diabetes published by the ADA. Or you can call the ADA at 800-232-6733 or visit the ADA website at www.diabetes.org to purchase books and publications about diabetes.

Many health professionals, such as nurses and registered dietitians (RDs), specialize in diabetes care and are called "certified diabetes educators" or CDEs. They have a wealth of information about diabetes. Ask your doctor to recommend a diabetes educator, or for a list of CDEs in your area, call the ADA at 800 DIABETES or the American Association of Diabetes Educators at 800 TEAM-UP-4.

27 Why do I yawn when I have low blood sugar?

Probably because low blood sugar makes you feel tired. The classic signs and symptoms of low blood sugar include sweating, hunger, nervousness, and agitation. However, some people experience no symptoms at all.

Other people have unusual symptoms of low blood sugar, including a change in personality, so that they become hostile and combative. Some people simply look glassy-eyed, "spacey," or are mildly confused. It is very important to know what your low blood-sugar symptoms are so that your friends and family will know when to help you.

28 Why do I always seem to get low blood sugar after having sex?

Sex is as much an exercise as jogging or aerobics. To avoid low blood sugar, eat food either immediately before or shortly after sex to replace the glucose that you use. You may want to check your blood sugar first, even though it may reduce the spontaneity of the moment. You might also consider increasing your snack before going to bed.

29 Why do I no longer feel the warning signs of low blood sugar?

Many people who have had diabetes for more than five years lose some of the symptoms of low blood sugar, a condition known as hypoglycemia unawareness. The usual feelings of hunger, sweatiness, anxiety, and increased heart rate may fade and escape your attention. Sometimes you may just feel sleepy as your blood-sugar level drops. The reasons for this are complex but are related to a loss of adrenaline release in your body when your blood sugar is low. If you are unaware of low blood sugars, try not to let your blood level drop below 100 mg/dl. You may need to monitor your blood-sugar levels more often, especially before you drive.

LIVING WELL—
DIET AND NUTRITION

30 How can I eat in a healthy way?

Ask your doctor to refer you to a registered dietitian (RD) who can design a meal plan tailored to your food likes and dislikes and your cooking ability. Try these tips:

- Eat more fresh (or frozen) vegetables and fruit daily.
- Eat more greens, like romaine, watercress, spinach, and arugula every day.
- Drink 6–8 glasses of water a day.
- Eat breakfast (try oatmeal).
- Eat an egg. It's a perfect food.
- For healthy fat, use olive oil to cook and add nuts to your oatmeal.
- Stop eating processed foods. (Read the ingredients—partially-hydrogenated oil is an unhealthy fat).

- Measure your servings with a measuring cup or food scale.
- Use herbs and spices instead of salt and fat.
- Buy a healthy cookbook.
- Stop smoking to improve your sense of taste and smell.

Think about the energy the food brings you and what you intend to do with the energy. Participate in the dance of life.

31 I've heard I'm supposed to eat five fruits and vegetables a day. Why?

Increasing fruits and vegetables in your diet gives you better health and helps prevent cancer and heart disease. Fruits and vegetables are low in fat and are rich sources of Vitamin A, Vitamin C, and fiber. The average American eats only one serving of fruit and two servings of vegetables a day. You can find ways to put five or more servings in your salads, soups, sandwiches, main dishes, and snacks.

Fruits and vegetables affect diabetes in different ways. Fruit has 15 grams of carbohydrates per serving. It affects your blood sugar within minutes, and those effects may last for two hours. The amount that blood sugar rises depends on whether you eat the fruit on an empty stomach, the form of the fruit (cooked or raw, whole or juice), and your blood-sugar level when you eat. Check your blood-sugar level after eating fruit to see what it does to you. Nonstarchy vegetables contain only 5 grams of carbohydrates per serving, few calories, and lots of vitamins and minerals. Moderate portions of non-starchy vegetables have little effect on blood sugar but major effects on your health. So eat up!

32 I don't have lots of time to spend shopping for food and making healthy meals. What can I do?

Here are some tips:

- Plan your meals for the week, using your diabetes meal plan as a guide. Do all your grocery shopping at once.
- Make a shopping list and move through the store quickly.
- Grated, chopped, precooked, and presliced foods save preparation time. For example, use prechopped broccoli florets from the salad bar.
- Cook once; serve two or three times. Plan to use leftovers. For example, if you are making pasta for a hot dish at supper, cook an extra handful to use in a cold pasta salad tomorrow. Make a pot roast with vegetables on Sunday and plan to use the leftover beef in beef stew, burritos, or vegetable-beef soup later in the week.
- Take a few minutes in the morning to assemble a slow-cooker recipe. Your reward: a ready-to-eat meal at the end of the day.
- Take advantage of the time you have on weekends. Cook and bake in large quantities and freeze portions for future meals and snacks.

33 How can I find a registered dietitian?

See a registered dietitian (RD) when your diabetes is first diagnosed, when a new doctor changes your treatment plan, or twice a year for a routine review of your meal plan and goals. See the RD more often if:

- You want to improve diabetes control.
- You experience lifestyle or schedule changes, such as a new job, marriage, or pregnancy.
- Your nutritional needs keep changing (this is true for children).
- You've begun an exercise program or had a change in diabetes medication.
- You feel bored, frustrated, or unmotivated to use your meal plan.
- You have unexplained high and low blood-sugar levels.
- You're concerned about weight or blood-fat levels.
- You've developed nutrition-related complications, such as high blood pressure or kidney disease.
- You're considering bariatric surgery.

We recommend having an RD on your diabetes team. Ask your doctor or hospital for a referral. You can call the American Diabetes Association (800-DIABETES), The American Dietetic Association (800-877-1600), or the American Association of Diabetes Educators (800-TEAM-UP-4) for referrals. Many RDs are certified diabetes educators (CDEs) and have additional training in diabetes care.

34 What is a meal plan?

Basically, a meal plan involves taking time to think about a meal before you eat it. Sometimes meal planning happens 10 minutes before your next meal; other times you can plan an entire week. No matter when it happens, an eating plan is an important part of diabetes therapy and can help you keep your blood sugars under control.

Meal plans can be tailored to fit your tastes and schedule, as well as your lifestyle. They help you manage the amount of carbohydrates and calories you take in on a daily basis. Meal planning is good if you have type 1 diabetes because you can match your insulin dose to the amount of carbohydrates you plan to eat. For type 2 diabetes, controlling the carbohydrates you take in can help keep your blood sugar in your target range.

35 I easily get overwhelmed with decisions. Would I do better if I had planned meals?

Yes. Studies have shown that people can achieve long-term success using menus or prepackaged foods. They help if you need more structure when starting a diet, when you are under stress, or when you have gained some weight.

Making food choices can be difficult when you are trying to break old habits. Using menus or packaged foods can make your decisions easier, because you can choose a cuisine and calorie level suited to your needs.

If you find yourself thinking, "I cannot wait until I finish this diet," you have a high risk of going back to your old habits. You may find that you will always need menus to keep you on track. If you use prepackaged meal supplements, make sure you don't round out the meal with high-calorie snacks. If you have a shake or a bar for one or two meals a day, you may find that you are hungry. Try to satisfy that hunger with raw vegetables or a piece of fruit as a snack.

36 Diet food and all those fruits and vegetables seem so expensive. How can following my meal plan cost less?

You can budget money as you are budgeting calories. You do not need to buy high-priced diet foods. Fresh fruits and vegetables and foods you prepare yourself are always the less expensive choice. You can choose to spend some time in order to save some money.

Low-calorie frozen entrées tend to cost more than the regular versions. Ones that have more meat cost more than the pasta-based entrées. Cutting down on high-priced meat can help save money that you can use to buy vegetables and fruits. Store brands of frozen vegetables are usually lower priced than national brands. When buying vegetables, compare the bagged ones with the ones you buy by the pound. Buying fruits in season can also save money—apples in the fall, citrus fruits in the winter, and berries in the spring.

Another way to save money is to buy produce directly from the farmer. The Web site for the United States Department of Agriculture (www.nal.usda.gov/afsic/csa/) provides information about the Community Supported Agriculture (CSA) program, which links local farmers to consumer buying groups whose members buy a share of the weekly harvest during the growing season.

37 How can I get my spouse to follow his or her meal plan?

There are many reasons your spouse might not follow the prescribed diet. First, he or she may not understand the meal plan. Did your spouse see a registered dietitian (RD) and receive easily understood written instructions describing the meal plan?

Second, your spouse may not believe that following it will work. Ask your spouse to try the prescribed diet for one month and measure weight and blood sugar daily to see what the effects are. Then he or she can decide whether the diet will help achieve his or her goals.

Third, your spouse may not want to eat foods that are different from those that the rest of the family eats. It helps if the whole family changes to a "diabetic" diet or meal plan, because it's a balanced, healthy diet that everyone should eat. Ask the RD to include some of your spouse's favorite foods into the meal plan.

Fourth, does your spouse understand the details of the diet? If you select and prepare the foods that your spouse eats, you also need to understand the meal plan and may want to discuss it with an RD.

Finally, remember that changing eating habits involves a lifestyle change, which is difficult for anyone. Don't try to change too many things too quickly. Your spouse will need support, understanding, and patience to achieve his or her goals.

38 How can keeping a food diary help my diabetes?

Until you write down the foods you eat, you probably are not aware of how much or what you are eating. A food diary helps you make important decisions about your medication, meal plan, and exercise plan. Following are tips for keeping a food diary.

Record information you need. If you want to lose weight, measure your serving sizes and write down how many calories or fat grams you're getting over several days. Looking up the nutrient values of foods helps you learn what nutrients each food gives you.

Keep records that are easy to use—a notebook, calendar, or form created on your computer. Write down what you eat and the time you eat it; don't wait until later. There are several apps available to help with this. Apps for keeping food diaries include MyFitness-Pal, MyNetDiary, LoseIt, and SparkPeople. A quick search will also yield several apps specifically for diabetes monitoring.

Use the information. Bring your record to the next appointment with your registered dietitian (RD). Look for patterns in your eating behaviors and blood-sugar levels. For example, your records may show that high-fat snacks in late afternoon result in high blood sugar at dinner. You may also notice that your lunch is much smaller than other meals, which causes you to feel too hungry before dinner. You may want to adjust the size of lunch and decrease your afternoon eating.

39 What is food combining and how does it work?

Several popular weight-loss diets recommend avoiding specific combinations of foods to improve digestion and metabolism. For example, some diets recommend that starchy foods be eaten alone to improve weight loss. People who go on these diets often do lose weight, but it's because they eat fewer calories and not necessarily because of the way foods are combined.

The food-combining approach encourages people to eat a lot of fruits and vegetables, a modest amount of starches, and limited portions of meat. Milk and dairy foods are not permitted at all. Each type of food is basically eaten alone, which reduces the tendency to overeat.

This structured approach does help avoid the added calories that come from unplanned eating. But you need very careful timing and planning to allow the recommended time to pass before eating a food that should not be combined with a previously eaten food. These dietary plans tend to be too low in calcium, Vitamin B12, Vitamin D, zinc, and protein.

40 Will becoming a vegetarian help my diabetes control?

Yes, a vegetarian diet can be a healthy choice for people with diabetes. There are several types of vegetarian diets.

- *Lacto-ovo-vegetarian*: eats no flesh foods, including meat, fish, seafood, poultry, or meat by-products, but consumes some dairy products and eggs.
- *Lacto-vegetarian*: eats no flesh foods, eggs, or meat by-products, but consumes some dairy products.
- *Vegan*: eats no foods of animal origin.

Vegetarian diets are based on fruits, vegetables, grains, beans, lentils, soybeans, nuts, and seeds. As a result, they are low in fat, cholesterol, and calories. Decreasing your use of animal products offers several diabetes health advantages. Vegetarians are less likely to be overweight, have high cholesterol levels, or have high blood pressure. They are also less likely to suffer from heart and blood vessel disease and certain cancers. If you have type 2 diabetes, the weight loss from a vegetarian diet may improve your blood-sugar control. A registered dietitian (RD) can help you plan vegetarian meals and ensure that you get all the vitamins, minerals, and protein you need.

41 How often do I need to eat for good diabetes control?

This depends on the type of diabetes you have, your medications, your physical activity, and your current blood-sugar level. A registered dietitian (RD) can help you decide.

For people with types 1 or 2 using insulin: Have food in your system when your insulin is peaking. You may need three meals and an evening snack. If you take two injections of short- and intermediate-acting insulin, you may need three meals and three snacks. If you use rapid-acting insulin, eat within 15 minutes of taking your insulin. You may need a snack for physical activity (see Tip 100 on page 125). A common mistake is not waiting a half hour to eat after taking regular insulin. If you start eating before insulin activity is peaking, you have higher blood-sugar levels after meals.

For type 2: Eat a small meal every two or three hours. When you eat smaller amounts of food, your blood-sugar levels are lower after eating. Mini-meals spread over the day may help control your hunger and calorie intake, leading to better blood-sugar control and weight loss. Your blood-cholesterol levels will also be lower.

42 Is it better to eat four or five small meals during the day instead of three large meals?

Yes! Scientists have been testing the ideal frequency of meals since the beginning of diabetes research. There are many benefits to eating small amounts of food over the course of the day rather than larger amounts at mealtimes. These benefits include decreased blood-sugar levels after a meal, reduced insulin requirements over the course of the day, and decreased blood-cholesterol levels. These benefits probably stem from a slow, continuous absorption of food from your gut, which spares your body the work of switching over to a "fasting" state. Also, eating several small meals a day may decrease your hunger and reduce the number of calories you eat.

Finally, there are diabetes medications available, such as acarbose, that slow the absorption of food and have much the same effect as eating your food slowly over the course of the day. The practice of nibbling may not appeal to everyone, but if it helps you maintain good blood-sugar control and a desirable body weight, then continue.

43 I'm not as hungry anymore, and I eat less often. Will this affect my diabetes control?

Yes. This is a change in your meal plan. If you use insulin, sulfonylureas, or meglitinides, not eating can put you at risk for very low blood sugar (hypoglycemia). Eating at odd times may give you wide swings in blood sugar and malnutrition. We do need less food as we age, but we still need to eat to stay healthy.

Perhaps you cannot taste or smell the food. Try brushing your tongue as well as your teeth before you eat. Stop smoking to improve your senses. Eat more fresh foods and use herbs and spices for flavor instead of salt.

Could you be depressed? Clinical depression is common in diabetes and certainly affects your appetite. Talk with your doctor about your symptoms. When you are depressed, it's difficult to be interested in doing things for yourself or staying healthy. It can keep you from getting up and going for a walk. Getting exercise will help build your appetite, improve your mental outlook, and give you more energy.

44 What foods can I eat when I am sick?

When you are sick, take your usual medication, check your blood sugar, and test your urine for ketones. If you can't eat regular food, consume carbohydrates in liquids or soft foods. Drink plenty of fluids—at least 4–6 ounces every hour. If you can't eat at your usual times, consume 15 grams of carbohydrates every hour to keep your blood sugar from dropping (see chart below).

These tips can help you handle sick days:

- Sip clear liquids, such as apple juice, sports drinks, or regular soda, if you can't keep anything else down.
- Use broth, vegetable juices, and sports drinks to replace potassium and sodium lost from diarrhea and vomiting.
- Ask your registered dietitian (RD) for sick-day meal plans.

Sick-Day Foods

15 grams of carbohydrates each	
1 cup broth soup	¼ cup sherbet
1 cup cream soup	½ cup regular soda
½ cup fruit juice	1 small frozen juice bar
1 cup milk or yogurt	1 cup sports drink
½ cup ice milk or ice cream	½ cup unsweetened applesauce
⅓ cup plain pudding	6 saltines
½ cup regular gelatin	

45 What can I eat for snacks?

Choose from the same healthy foods that you eat at meals, foods with 15 grams of carbohydrates per serving. Choose foods from the grain group, such as air-popped popcorn, baked tortilla chips and salsa, graham crackers, pretzels, bagels, or cereal. Fresh fruits and vegetables make excellent snacks, and they're also portable. To make a snack more substantial, add a source of low-fat protein, such as low-fat milk, reduced-fat peanut butter on a slice of bread or a bagel, low-fat cheese on crackers, or a slice of turkey breast on whole-wheat bread.

Be prepared! Always carry a snack with you in case of a delayed meal or an unexpected change in your schedule. Snacks can be stashed in your desk, briefcase, backpack, or glove compartment. Having good food on hand will save you from hypoglycemia and from having to settle for less nutritious fast-foods.

46 Does reading food labels help me stay healthy?

Yes. Food labels provide important information that can help you eat healthy meals and snacks. Food and Drug Administration (FDA) regulations require all food labels to include:

- The standard serving size
- Total calories, and calories from fat in each serving
- A list of nutrients and ingredients
- The recommended daily amounts of nutrients in the food
- The relationship between the food and any disease it may affect

Make a habit of reading food labels and become familiar with the amount of calories, fats, carbohydrates, and sodium in them. For many foods, you have a choice of different brands, and by comparing food labels, you can choose the healthiest brand. Food label information helps you keep track of the amount of nutrients you eat daily, which is vital to a healthy diet.

47 How big is a serving?

This is tricky to answer. Good nutrition comes in many different shapes and sizes, and it may be difficult to determine the appropriate serving size for various foods and liquids. The USDA gives a wide range of servings from each of the six major food groups. However, serving sizes are different within each group, and from group to group.

Serving sizes are used to keep the level of calories, carbohydrates, protein, and fat the same within each group. When calories and carbohydrates are the same for each meal, day to day, then it's easier to keep your blood sugar stable. Below is a list of some serving sizes.

- 1 slice bread
- ½ cup cooked cereal
- ½ cup cooked rice or pasta
- ½ cup cooked legumes
- 1 cup milk or yogurt
- 1½ oz cheese
- 1 cup raw, leafy vegetables
- ½ cup cooked starchy vegetables
- ¾ cup vegetable juice
- 1 medium-size apple, banana, orange, or pear
- ½ cup fruit chopped, cooked, or canned in water
- ½ cup fruit juice
- 2-3 oz cooked beef, poultry, or fish
- 1 egg

48   Why are serving sizes important? Is there an easy way to remember them?

No matter which meal plan you follow—carbohydrate-counting, exchanges, or the Food Guide Pyramid—serving size is key. An extra ounce of meat or tablespoon of margarine doesn't sound like much, but it can quickly add up to higher blood-sugar levels and weight gain.

Begin by using standard kitchen measuring cups, spoons, and food scales until you train your eyes to see correct serving sizes. Once you've weighed, measured, and looked at a half cup of green beans or 5 ounces of chicken, you'll have a mental picture no matter where you dine. Every few months, measure some servings again to keep your eyes sharp and your servings the right size. The following chart lists the serving sizes of various foods.

Serving Sizes at a Glance

Food	Looks Like
½ cup cooked pasta or rice	a baseball
½ cup vegetables	half a tennis ball
1 cup broccoli	a light bulb
3 oz meat, chicken, or fish	a deck of cards or the palm of a woman's hand
1 oz cheese	two saltine crackers or a 1-inch square cube

49 How many grams of sugar am I allowed to eat in a day?

There is no magic number of grams for each day, but eat sugar sparingly. Sugar has calories but few vitamins or minerals. Foods high in sugar are usually also high in fat and calories, which can lead to poor diabetes control and weight gain.

The Nutrition Facts label on packaging gives the number of grams of sugar in the food. This number includes both natural and added sugars. Natural sugars are found naturally in foods, such as fructose in raisins or lactose in milk. These sugars provide some vitamins and minerals. Added sugars are put into foods to make them sweet, such as sugar in cookies or high-fructose corn syrup in soft drinks. These sugars provide calories but no other nutrients.

When you read the food label, check the type of sugar the food contains, but focus on the grams of total carbohydrates rather than the grams of sugar. Sugar and sweets are fine occasionally and in small portions. The key is to substitute them for other carbohydrate foods in your meal plan and check your blood sugar to see how the food affects you.

50 Now that sugar is no longer forbidden for people with diabetes, can I eat all the sweets I want?

It's true that the carbohydrate in table sugar generally has the same effect on your blood sugar as any other carbohydrate, such as that in bread, potatoes, or fruit. Different carbohydrates raise blood sugar in different ways; however, for blood-sugar control, it's more important to focus on the total amount of carbohydrates you eat rather than their source. Substitute sweets into your meal plan for other carbohydrates—don't add them on top.

And don't have sweets at every meal. Sugary foods don't have the nutrients, vitamins, and minerals that your body needs to be healthy, which is why we call these calories "empty." If you include sweets in a meal, eat a small serving and check your blood sugar before you eat, and between one and two hours after, to see how it affects you. Keep an eye on your weight and blood-sugar levels over time, and hold back on the sweets if you see your numbers creeping up.

51 I'm confused about sugars and starches. Which raises my blood sugar more— a brownie or a piece of bread?

Sugars and starches are carbohydrates and, eaten in equal amounts, they raise blood sugar about the same. A small brownie (15 grams of carbohydrates) raises blood sugar the same as one slice of bread (15 grams of carbohydrates).

For years, we thought that the body absorbed sugar more quickly than starch, and people were told to avoid sweets. Certain carbohydrates are absorbed at different rates, but when combined with other foods in a meal, this effect can be hard to predict. Research has shown that sugar is okay for people with diabetes if it is part of a meal plan, but it must be substituted for other carbohydrate foods. Focus on the total amount of carbohydrates that you eat rather than on whether it comes from starch or sugar.

Certain factors affect the way your blood sugar responds to sugars and starches. When you eat sweets, observe whether other foods are eaten at the same time, how quickly you eat, how the food was prepared (baked, fried, etc.), and the amount of protein and fat in the food. Measure your blood sugar between one and two hours after eating and note the effect sugar has on it. Use this information to track your food habits and preferences and to make decisions about including sweets in your meal plan.

52 Are there sweeteners that are "free foods"? How can I tell which to use?

Nonnutritive sweeteners are free foods because they have no calories or carbohydrates. They also don't raise blood-sugar levels. ("Free food" is a term used by people with diabetes for foods that have less than 20 calories or less than 5 grams of carbohydrates per serving.) None of these nonnutritive sweeteners are perfect for all uses (see chart below). Some are great in cold beverages but won't work in baked goods. While the sweeteners themselves are calorie-free, don't forget to count the calories, fat, and carbohydrates in the foods they are sweetening.

Nonnutritive Sweeteners and Their Uses

Sweetener (brands)	Calories (per gram)	Description
Saccharin (*Sweet'N Low*)	0	200–700 times sweeter than sucrose; suitable for cooking and baking
Aspartame (*Nutrasweet, Equal*)	0	160–220 times sweeter than sucrose; may change flavor; suitable for sweetening prepared foods such as cereal or beverages; not suitable for cooking
Acesulfame (*Sunette, Sweet One*)	0	200 times sweeter than sucrose; suitable for cooking
Sucralose (*Splenda*)	0	600 times sweeter than sucrose; suitable for cooking and baking

53 Can I eat all I want of food that is labeled sugar-free?

No. A food labeled sugar-free must contain less than 0.5 grams of sugar per serving, but it may have calories and carbohydrates. For example, sugar-free pudding has 0 grams of sugar, but it also has 70 calories and 6 grams of carbohydrates in a half-cup serving. If you were to eat unlimited amounts, you could easily add enough calories and carbohydrates to sabotage your diabetes and weight-control efforts over time.

Some sugar alcohols will not raise your blood sugar levels but can have other negative side effects. For example, for some people even small amounts of sorbitol or manitol may cause diarrhea. Other sugar alcohols, like erythritol, don't seem to have this negative effect, but each body is different, so try a small amount of a sugar alcohol to see how you react before consuming more.

Although the sweetener used in a sugar-free product may be calorie-free (such as acesulfame potassium, aspartame, saccharin, or sucralose), the other ingredients in the food usually contain fat, carbohydrates, protein, and calories. Other sweeteners that contain calories may be used along with the nonnutritive sweetener, so don't rely on the sugar-free symbol on the package. Read the ingredient list and food label carefully so you can make the best choices for healthy eating.

54 Why do some sugar-free foods taste weird?

While some foods are actually improved by becoming sugar-free (canned fruit, for example), other foods are not so successfully converted to sugar-free. These are usually foods in which artificial sweeteners (sorbitol, saccharin, or aspartame) are added. But these sweeteners do not cook like sugar, so they don't work well in baked foods and may leave a bitter aftertaste. Also, remember that these foods are not necessarily low in calories. For example, sugar-free pudding made with reduced-fat milk has 90 calories per serving as compared to 140 calories per serving for regular pudding. Although 90 is less than 140, it still isn't calorie-free. You don't have to eat only sugar-free cookies. You may have a real cookie—just include it in your meal plan.

55 How can I overcome my craving for chocolate?

Give in once in a while! By denying your desire for chocolate (or any other particular food), you are setting yourself up for failure. If you find yourself craving a food and expending effort to avoid it, you may eventually give up and overindulge. Then your blood-sugar control suffers, and you feel guilty and depressed.

Think about some healthy ways to satisfy your craving. For chocolate lovers, dark or bitter chocolate is preferred to milk chocolate, which has higher dairy fat. We suggest low-fat frozen yogurt. It tastes great, has less than 1 gram of fat, and is inexpensive. Another treat is chocolate graham crackers, which may also be used for making desserts. Make a fancy dessert with angel-food cake, strawberries, and chocolate syrup. Yes, the syrup has some sugar in it, but it is almost fat-free. Whether you have type 1 or type 2 diabetes, fat is a critical concern and is actually the worst part of most candies.

Recent research has shown that sugar has about the same effect on your blood sugar as an equal amount of carbohydrates from potatoes or rice. So when you must have chocolate, choose a relatively low-fat variety and substitute it into your meal plan for other carbohydrates.

56 Should I use fructose as a sweetener when I bake?

Fructose is not necessarily better for you than plain sugar. Fructose is a naturally occurring sweetener like table sugar (sucrose). It may produce a smaller rise in blood sugar than the same number of calories of table sugar. This is good for people with diabetes; however, large amounts of fructose can increase your total cholesterol and bad cholesterol (LDL) levels. That's why fructose is really no better for you than other sugars. People with abnormally high or low blood-cholesterol levels should avoid consuming large amounts of fructose.

57 Why is fat in food so bad?

Fats are not the root of all evil. In fact, fats:

- help your body and brain work
- transport essential vitamins (A, D, and E)
- make skin and hair look healthy
- reduce hunger feelings
- make food taste good

But too much of a good thing is bad. Excessive amounts of fat in your diet are linked to a variety of health issues. This is especially true as you age. Excessive amounts of fat in your bloodstream can stick to your arteries, causing them to constrict blood flow. When you have diabetes, these fats become stickier and cause even more buildup. The buildup increases with age, narrowing your arteries, too. When the space inside your arteries shrinks, you develop high blood pressure (hypertension), and a higher risk for heart attack and stroke.

When you eat wisely, choosing healthier fats such as olive oil instead of butter or margarine (or even dark chocolate instead of milk chocolate), and cut some processed or fried foods out of your meal plan, you significantly reduce the risks to your health.

58 How do I know if I'm eating the right amount of fat?

Talk to a registered dietitian (RD) about the right amount of fat for you, based on your weight and blood-sugar and lipid goals. Most people eat too much fat. Fats contain nine calories per gram, which means they contain a lot of calories in a small amount of food.

Write down what you eat for a few days, including the fat grams in your foods. The Nutrition Facts panel on food labels gives this information. For most people, fat should contribute about 30% of total calories for the day. Here is how to figure the number of grams of fat to eat if 30% of your 1,800 calories come from fat:

To find 30% of 1,800 calories:
1,800 x 0.30 = 540 calories from fat

To find the number of fat grams in 540 calories
(9 calories per 1 gram of fat):
540 ÷ 9 = 60 grams of fat per day

Calories/Fat Conversion

Total Calories	Fat (g) for 30% of Calories
1,200	40
1,500	50
1,800	60
2,100	70
2,400	80
2,600	87

59 How can I make my favorite recipes lower in fat?

These tips may help:

Most recipes (except some baked goods) will taste fine if you reduce the butter or oil by one-third or one-half. When baking, substitute two egg whites for a whole egg; use fat-free milk instead of whole milk. Reduced-calorie butter or margarine has too much water to use for baking. Because fat gives texture to baked goods, decreasing it can be tricky. Try replacing oil, margarine, or butter with applesauce. Use an equal amount of fruit for fat to retain moisture and flavor. Puréed prunes taste great in chocolate desserts.

Marinades need acid, such as lemon juice, vinegar, or wine, more than oil for tenderizing.

Use lower-fat substitutes. Low-fat yogurt replaces sour cream in dips and dressings. Use evaporated fat-free milk instead of heavy cream. Replace half the ground meat in casseroles with mashed beans or cooked brown rice. Use butter-flavored spray on cooked vegetables, baked potatoes, or popcorn.

Cocoa powder gives chocolate flavor without the fat. When baking use 3 tablespoons unsweetened cocoa powder and 1 tablespoon olive or coconut oil to replace 1 ounce unsweetened chocolate.

60 What are fat replacers?

Fat replacers are ingredients that manufacturers put in food to mimic the attributes of fat while reducing fat and calories. These replacers can be made of carbohydrates, protein, or fat. Fat replacers may be advantageous to your diet because fat contains 9 calories per gram of food, a very high energy content for a small amount of food. Many fat replacers, particularly if they are carbohydate- and protein-based, contain only 5 calories per gram of food. So, if you eat the same weight of food, you actually get half as many calories and might, therefore, lose weight.

The problem is that many people assume that fat-free foods are much lower in calories than they are, and they eat much larger servings of them. Fat-free does not mean calorie-free. Also, watch for fat replacers that are made of carbohydrates because they will affect your blood-sugar level.

61 Can I eat an unlimited amount of fat-free foods?

No. Fat-free does not mean the food is calorie-free or carbohydrate-free. Nor does it mean that it is a "free food." Free foods have less than 20 calories or less than 5 grams of carbohydrates per serving.

Fat-free foods have fat taken out and sometimes replaced by fat replacers. Some fat replacers, such as those used in fat-free salad dressings, contain carbohydrates and can affect your blood-sugar level. Also, many fat-free foods have sugar added for taste, and this will affect your blood-sugar level.

If your weight and blood lipids are in a healthy range, you don't need fat-free foods. If your goal is to lower blood lipids and lose weight, moderate portions of some fat-free foods may help you. Read the Nutrition Facts on food labels to get the serving size, calories, and carbohydrate content to help you decide how fat-free foods fit into your meal plan.

62 What are trans fatty acids and how do they affect my diabetes?

Trans fatty acids are formed in processed foods during hydrogenation. Hydrogenation makes a fat solid when it is at room temperature. For example, liquid vegetable oil is partially hydrogenated to make stick margarine. Partially hydrogenated vegetable oil is used in fried foods, baked products, and snack foods. As of January 2006, food manufacturers were required to list trans fats on the Nutrition Facts label of food products.

Trans fatty acids don't affect blood-sugar levels but do increase blood-cholesterol levels, which raises your risk for heart disease. If less than 30% of your calories come from fat and 10% from saturated fat, you're probably okay. If you eat a moderately high-fat diet, your trans fatty acid intake may be too high. Avoid processed foods. Choose soft table spreads instead of stick margarine. Read food labels and select margarine that contains no more than 2 grams of saturated fat per tablespoon, and liquid oil as the first ingredient. Look for baked products, convenience dinners, and snack foods with less than 2 grams of saturated fat per serving. Use vegetable oil instead of solid shortening in cooking. Check with your registered dietitian (RD) if you have questions about trans fatty acids.

63 What are omega-3 fatty acids and should I include them in my diet?

Research has indicated that omega-3 fatty acids play a role in healthier diets. These fats have a different chemical structure than other fats. They improve good cholesterol (HDL) and improve blood flow by making your blood cells less "sticky." A diet high in omega-3 fatty acids can lower your risk of heart attack and various other heart problems, and lower your risk of stroke. It also can lower triglyceride levels and slightly reduce an elevated blood pressure.

Because foods high in omega-3 fatty acids tend to be high in fat, they should replace other fatty foods in your diet. Omega-3 fatty acids can be found in fish, such as mackerel, herring, sardines, salmon, and trout. The best plant sources for omega-3 fatty acids are tofu, soybean oil, canola oil, and nuts. Fish oil supplements containing omega-3 fatty acids are also available, but it is better to eat a healthy diet than to add supplements.

64 How can I eat my favorite foods when dining out?

Successful weight managers advise, "If you want it, have it." Try to break away from good food/bad food thinking. Instead, when you have treats, enjoy them — and don't feel guilty. But plan, plan, plan. For, "If you fail to plan, you plan to fail."

Identify the food that is important to you and figure how many calories are in the serving you require to enjoy that food. Using that calorie amount, figure what else can be included in the meal, if anything. Add the total calories you need to save up for the treat. Figure what your usual calories would be at that meal, and subtract them from the calories in the treat meal. For example, if you usually eat 450 calories at lunch, but your favorite food is 950 calories, you have 500 extra calories to deduct from your week. Don't try to take the 500 calories from the other meals in that same day. It's better to cut some calories each day for several days before the treat. And remember that you can burn calories with exercise, too. Everything counts.

65 How can I reduce fat in a meal when I eat at a restaurant?

First identify your habits by answering these questions:

- How often do you eat out?
- What meals do you eat out most often?
- What type of restaurants do you choose most often?
- What foods do you order?

Knowing these details about your eating habits can help pinpoint poor eating choices and change them. Select restaurants that offer lower-fat choices. Get copies of menus and decide what you will eat before you arrive. Plan ways to balance your restaurant meal with food choices the rest of the day. Save fat choices for your meal out.

When ordering, meat is the best place to start cutting fat calories. The best choices are grilled, baked, braised, broiled, poached, roasted, steamed, or stir-fried. Fish that is broiled or baked usually has less than 5 grams of fat per ounce. When ordering beef, look for a lower-fat cut, such as sirloin, instead of prime rib or filet. Ask how many ounces are in the serving size. You may even request a smaller serving, such as "a 4-ounce serving of the sirloin," or request that the meat be prepared with no fat. Meats that are processed, such as bratwurst, lunch meats, and sausages, can be very high in fat—between 10 and 15 grams per ounce—and are usually very high in salt as well.

Avoid foods that are fried, breaded, buttered, creamed, sautéed, scalloped, or served with gravy or a thick sauce. Ask about food preparation and ingredients, and request that sauces and salad dressings be served on the side. Decline any extra bread or tortilla chips.

If a serving seems too big, order an appetizer instead, split a main dish with your dining companion, or take home leftovers. Set aside the portion you want to take home as soon as the food arrives.

66 Will fiber help my diabetes control?

Fiber can keep your blood sugar from spiking after a meal because it slows down the speed at which food is digested. A high-fiber, low-fat diet can also reduce your risk of cancer, cardiovascular disease, high blood pressure, and obesity. Fiber has a favorable effect on cholesterol, too.

There are two types of fiber in foods: insoluble fiber, such as that in vegetables and whole-grain products, and soluble fiber, found in fruits, oats, barley, and beans. Insoluble fiber improves gastrointestinal function, including preventing hemorrhoids, diverticulosis, and colon and rectal cancer. In large amounts, soluble fiber can prevent your body from absorbing glucose and cholesterol. Unfortunately, most Americans eat only 8–10 grams of fiber daily, not the recommended 20–35 grams a day from a variety of foods. You can increase fiber by eating foods such as the ones in the chart on page 89. Another way to increase fiber in your diet is to take a tablespoon of pseudophilin (Metamucil) at bedtime.

Fiber-Rich Foods (grams per serving)

Food	Serving Size	Total Fiber (g)	Soluble Fiber (g)
Beans	½ cup cooked	6.9	2.8
Oat Bran	⅓ cup dry	4.0	2.0
Barley	¼ cup dry	3.0	0.9
Orange, fresh	1 small	2.9	1.8
Oatmeal	⅓ cup dry	2.7	1.4

If you count carbs and there are more than 5 grams of fiber in the serving you eat, subtract the number of grams of fiber from the grams of total carbohydrates. Use that number for the carb count in the food. The carbs from fiber will not raise your blood sugar. (For more on counting carbohydrates, see Tip 68 on page 91.)

67 Is it true that beans can improve diabetes control?

Yes. Legumes are very high in carbohydrates and need to be eaten in the proper portions, but because they digest slowly, they raise blood-sugar and insulin levels minimally. Several research studies have shown that eating 1½-2½ cups of cooked beans daily helps control diabetes. Beans also reduce the risk of cardio-vascular disease, a common complication for people with diabetes. Eating 1-3 cups of cooked beans a day will lower total cholesterol by 5-19%. Beans are also an excellent source of folate, which may reduce the risk of cardiovascular disease.

Packed with protein, fiber, vitamins, and minerals, beans are also low in fat, cholesterol, and sodium. They can be included in all types of diabetes meal plans, including salads, soups, or entrées. Canned beans require less preparation time and have the same beneficial effects as dried beans, which require soaking and rinsing well before cooking. It's important to introduce beans gradually into your diet, chew thoroughly, and drink plenty of liquids to aid digestion. Enzyme products such as Beano can also help you avoid gastrointestinal distress.

68 What is carbohydrate counting?

This is a precise method of meal planning for people with diabetes. Foods containing carbohydrates (grains, vegetables, fruit, milk, and sugar) have the largest effect on blood-sugar level. A small amount of carbohydrates (one apple) raises blood sugar some; a larger amount of carbohydrates (three apples) raises blood sugar more. You track how the carbohydrates affect you by monitoring your blood sugar. You have to invest some time in monitoring blood sugar, record-keeping, measuring food servings, and learning about nutrients in foods.

Carbohydrate counting has two levels: basic and advanced. Basic carbohydrate counting is generally used by people with type 2 diabetes and consists mostly of counting and eating consistent amounts of carbohydrates. Advanced is often used by people taking insulin and is made up of recognizing and managing patterns in blood-sugar levels, food consumption, medication, and exercise for intensive management of blood sugar. You may only need to learn about basic carbohydrate counting. The amount of work may seem overwhelming at first, but most people find that the improvements in blood-sugar control are worth it! A registered dietitian (RD) can help you learn carbohydrate counting.

69 Is protein good for me?

Protein is good for your health, but most Americans get more than they need. If just 10% of your calories come from protein, this is usually enough for your body's needs.

Protein is found in many foods but is particularly high in meat, dairy products, and eggs. Talk to your diabetes care team to create an individualized goal for protein consumption.

70 Are plant sources of protein better for me than animal protein?

Maybe. Plant proteins have benefits for people with diabetes. Plant foods are low in fat, especially saturated fat, and high in fiber. Animal protein adds cholesterol and saturated fat to our diets. People with diabetes have a greater risk of heart disease earlier in life; therefore it is important to decrease saturated fat and cholesterol.

For people with diabetic kidney disease, changing the source of protein in the diet as a treatment is being studied. Whether plant proteins (beans, nuts, vegetables, tofu) are preferred over animal proteins (meat, poultry, fish, milk, eggs) has not been decided. Discuss the latest research with your diabetes professionals. We do know that people in other countries who eat less meat and more soy protein and rice have fewer cancers and heart disease than Americans who eat lots of animal protein.

Animal protein contains all eight essential amino acids that you need to build cells in the body. Because your body can't make them, your food choices must supply them. However, eating a variety of plant proteins each day can also provide all the amino acids that you need.

71 Are eggs off-limits now that I have diabetes?

No. Contrary to the widely-held belief that cholesterol-rich eggs are bad for heart health, several research studies have found that for most people, dietary cholesterol has little effect on the cholesterol level in blood. Saturated fat has a more significant effect on your blood-cholesterol level (see Tip 77 on pages 101-102). A person's response to dietary cholesterol is highly individual and genetically determined. About 20% of us have little or no response to dietary cholesterol; 50% show a small response; and the remaining 30% are responders, particularly sensitive to high-cholesterol foods. There is no easy test to determine who is cholesterol sensitive, so just be cautious when using eggs and other cholesterol-rich foods.

An egg is an economical source of protein, providing 70 calories, less than 1 gram of carbohydrates, 4.5 grams of fat, and 1 gram of saturated fat. One egg contains vitamins, minerals, and about 215 mg of cholesterol.

Don't eliminate eggs from your diet. Use them wisely or follow the American Heart Association guideline — no more than four a week.

72   How can I use herbs and spices?

Herbs and spices taste good, smell good, and best of all, have no effect on diabetes control. They are "free foods" on every meal plan. Herbs and spices come fresh or dried. Dried herbs have more intense flavor. (When substituting fresh for dried herbs, double or triple the amount.) The amount of herb or spice that you use in a recipe depends on individual taste.

Try these traditional pairings to "spice up" your meal:

- Beef: bay leaf, chives, garlic, marjoram, savory
- Lamb: garlic, marjoram, mint, oregano, rosemary, sage, savory
- Pork: cilantro, cumin, ginger, sage, thyme
- Poultry: garlic, oregano, rosemary, sage, thyme
- Seafood: chervil, dill weed, fennel, tarragon, parsley
- Pasta: basil, oregano, fennel, garlic, paprika, parsley, sage
- Rice: marjoram, parsley, tarragon, thyme, turmeric
- Potatoes: chives, garlic, paprika, parsley, rosemary
- Fruits: cinnamon, cloves, ginger, mint
- Salads: basil, chervil, chives, dill weed, marjoram, mint, oregano, parsley, tarragon, thyme

Be aware that some herb blends contain sodium, such as lemon pepper, or are salts, such as garlic salt.

73 Are sports drinks such as Gatorade okay for people with diabetes?

Yes, but be careful. Some sports drinks have a lot of sugar and could affect your blood sugar in nasty ways. Not having enough fluid during or after exercise can lead to serious problems, so drinking plenty of fluids is important. Drink at least two quarts of fluid a day to avoid dehydration. Drinking an extra 4–8 ounces of fluid for each 30 minutes of intense exercise will help your body achieve peak performance and recovery. Drinking something other than water can add variety, but sports drinks contain about 15–20 grams of sugar and 50–70 calories per 8 ounces, and the sugar is often in the form of fructose corn syrup.

Take the time to read labels and compare ingredients, sugar, and carbohydrate amounts before drinking these products. Always check blood-sugar levels before and after exercise. Listed below are some sports drinks and the grams of sugar and calories for each.

Sports Drinks' Calorie/Sugar Content

Sports Drink	Calories	Sugar (in grams)
All Sport 8 oz	70	19 g
Gatorade 8 oz	50	14 g
Powerade 8 oz	70	15 g

74 Is it acceptable for me to have a drink with dinner?

It may be. Alcohol can cause severe, life-threatening low blood sugar, even in people who do not have diabetes. That is why we suggest drinking alcohol *only with food*. Evidence shows that small amounts of alcohol are okay for people with diabetes who are not pregnant and have no history of alcohol abuse.

For example, one study shows that moderate alcohol intake (no more than one drink a day) is associated with lower blood-sugar levels and improved insulin sensitivity in healthy people who do not have diabetes. Another study shows that blood-sugar levels do not differ for 12 hours following a meal between diabetes patients (both types 1 and 2) who drink a shot of vodka before dinner, *or* a glass of wine with dinner, *or* a shot of cognac after dinner, and those who drink an equal amount of water.

Finally, a number of studies suggest that moderate alcohol intake may have a positive effect on blood-cholesterol and lipid levels. Just remember to include alcohol calories in your meal plan (one alcoholic drink is 1 fat exchange) and enjoy your one drink with food. Do not drink any alcohol if you are taking Metformin, and remember that binge drinking increases the risk for lactic acidosis, the buildup of lactic acid in the bloodstream.

LIVING WELL—
MATTERS OF THE HEART

75 Am I at more risk to develop heart disease because I have diabetes?

Yes. For unknown reasons, having diabetes puts you at an increased risk of heart disease and other diseases that are caused by blocked arteries. In fact, your risk is the same as a person without diabetes who has had one heart attack. Therefore it is very important to minimize your other risk factors by getting plenty of exercise, keeping your weight normal, avoiding fatty foods (saturated fat), and maintaining normal blood pressure. Walking is good exercise and helps in all those areas and reduces stress.

Most important, in our opinion, is that you do not smoke. If you are already smoking, join a "quit smoking" support group. These are available in most communities and health-care facilities. Nicotine skin patches also may help. Many of the risk factors that cause heart disease can be reduced significantly with a healthy lifestyle, and this should be your goal with or without diabetes. However, because you already have one risk factor for heart disease (diabetes), there is even more reason to reduce other risk factors.

76 How high is my risk for heart attack with type 2 diabetes?

Higher than you might think! One study found that people with type 2 diabetes, who have not had a heart attack, have as high a risk for a future heart attack as a person without diabetes who has already had a heart attack. In other words, your risk for a future heart attack is the same as the risk for a person without diabetes who has known heart disease.

This finding suggests that risk factors for heart disease, such as smoking, high blood pressure, and high blood-cholesterol levels, should be treated very aggressively in people with diabetes. Some experts even recommend that people with type 2 diabetes take medication as if they already have heart disease. So if your diabetes-care team suggests specific treatment to lower your risk of heart attack, you should strongly consider giving it a try.

77 Will lowering the fat in my diet reduce my risk for heart disease?

In most cases, yes. You will especially lower your risk if you lower the saturated fats. Fats fall into one of three groups.

Saturated fat: Increases total cholesterol in your blood and the risk of heart disease. These fats are usually solid at room temperature and are found in animal fats (meat, butter, lard, bacon, cheese); coconut, palm, and palm kernel oils; dairy fats; and hydrogenated vegetable fats, such as vegetable shortening and stick margarine.

Monounsaturated fat: Lowers total cholesterol, does not affect HDL (good) levels, and may reduce triglyceride levels. Food sources are olive oil, peanut oil, canola oil, olives, avocados, and nuts (except walnuts, which are polyunsaturated).

Polyunsaturated fat: Lowers total cholesterol levels but may also lower HDL (good) levels. Food sources are vegetable oils, such as corn, safflower, soybean, sunflower, and cottonseed.

The chart on page 102 summarizes the effects of these fats.

Types of Fats and Their Effects

Type of Fat	Effect on Your Body	Net Effect
Saturated fat: animal fats, lard	Increases total cholesterol, increases heart disease	✗
Monounsaturated fat: olive oil, canola oil, nuts, avocados	Lowers total cholesterol, no effect on HDL (good cholesterol)	✓
Polyunsaturated fat: corn oil, safflower oil	Lowers total cholesterol, positive and negative effect on HDL	✓

78 What is the difference between "good" and "bad" cholesterol?

The target for cholesterol in adults is less than 100 mg/dl of low-density lipoprotein. The ADA recommends that people with diabetes have blood lipids checked every year. A lipid profile measures the levels of high-density lipoprotein (HDL), low-density lipoprotein (LDL), and triglycerides.

HDL (good) cholesterol carries cholesterol from every part of the body back to the liver for disposal. If you have high levels of HDL cholesterol (higher than 40 mg/dl for men, 50 mg/dl for women), you are less likely to have heart disease.

LDL (bad) cholesterol carries cholesterol from the liver to other tissues. Along the way, it forms deposits on the walls of arteries and other blood vessels. High levels of LDL cholesterol (above 100 mg/dl) show an increased risk of heart disease. Your body stores extra fat and calories as triglycerides. Good triglyceride levels are less than 200 mg/dl.

79 How much can changes in diet lower my blood-cholesterol level?

Diet changes may decrease your LDL (bad) cholesterol by 15–25 mg/dl. For every 1% decrease in your total cholesterol, you decrease your risk for heart disease by 2%. Wouldn't you rather improve your risk factors for heart disease without medications, using diet changes only?

A heart-healthy eating plan is low in saturated fat and dietary cholesterol, with total fat around 30% of total calories. This helps reduce blood cholesterol. Eating foods containing more fiber, such as beans, can also help reduce blood levels of cholesterol (see Tip 66 on pages 88-89). A registered dietitian (RD) can help you find the best amounts of fats, carbohydrates, and proteins in your food choices to lower your cholesterol, maintain healthy weight, and have good blood-sugar control.

The following suggestions can help you eat low-fat meals:

- Select lean meats and cook with little or no fat.
- Choose low-fat or fat-free milk products.
- Eat less meat, cheese, and bacon.
- Eat low-fat breads and starchy foods, such as potatoes, rice, and beans.

Remember that sweets, such as pastries and chocolate, are often also high in fat.

80 Why did my doctor recently start me on a blood-pressure medication even though my blood pressure is only slightly elevated?

High blood sugar combined with high blood pressure increases your risk of getting diabetic kidney disease. Kidney disease can lead to kidney failure and the need for either dialysis or a kidney transplant. Doctors can identify diabetic kidney disease at a very early stage, when small amounts of protein (microalbuminuria) appear in the urine. Certain drugs that lower blood pressure, such as ACE inhibitors, also lower microalbuminuria and can slow the development of kidney disease.

81 What diet change must I make to improve my blood pressure?

If you are sensitive to sodium, lowering the sodium in your diet may make a big difference in your blood pressure. Less sodium in your body means you retain less water, have less fluid in your blood vessels, and less "pressure" in your system. Sodium is a major part of table salt. Sodium is also used as a preservative and flavor enhancer in foods that may not even taste salty. Try these tips to lower your sodium intake:

1. Always taste your food before reaching for the salt shaker.
2. Use pepper and other seasonings to add flavor before adding salt.
3. Cook with a variety of seasonings, such as onion and garlic.
4. Add a dash of lemon juice to vegetables and salads to brighten the flavor.
5. Avoid seasoned salt or garlic salt; use garlic powder or fresh garlic.
6. Try a commercial salt-free seasoning mix and carry a small container of it with you.
7. Ask for foods to be prepared without salt in restaurants and ask for sauces on the side.
8. Read the labels on prepared foods and canned goods to avoid high-salt items, and find no-salt-added or low-sodium products.

Remember, the closer to nature a food is, the more likely it will be low in salt.

LIVING WELL—
WEIGHT MANAGEMENT
AND EXERCISE

82 How does losing weight improve my health?

Losing weight can reduce your risk of getting diabetes, heart disease, high blood pressure, gallbladder disease, and breast and colon cancer. If you already have any of these health problems, losing weight improves them. When you lose weight, you'll spend less time and money on doctor's visits and treating health problems.

People who lose even small amounts of weight—5-7% of their starting weight (usually 10-20 pounds)—improve their health by reducing high blood pressure, blood sugar, and cholesterol. Losing weight also improves sleep apnea, arthritis, depression, and self-esteem. Even without weight loss, you enjoy health benefits as soon as you take steps to improve your lifestyle with a meal plan and more physical activity. Just do it.

83 Should I join an expensive diet and weight-reduction program to lose weight?

We don't recommend it. You will probably waste your time and money. Advertisements for these programs usually show before and after photographs of heavy people who have lost weight. What these advertisements don't show are the people who never lost a pound. More importantly, long-term studies show that almost everyone who loses weight rapidly over several months gains it all back by the end of five years. Also, very low-calorie diets can be dangerous, because they can cause serious chemical imbalances and vitamin deficiencies.

A much better plan to lose weight is to make small changes in your lifestyle, so that you lose between one-half and one pound per month. Over five years, this small change equals a 50-pound weight loss! In comparison to expensive diet programs, low-cost weight-reduction programs, such as Weight Watchers or TOPS (Take Off Pounds Sensibly), can provide much support and advice for you. In addition, your health-care team can be a great help in suggesting ways to make small but positive changes in your lifestyle to accomplish your weight goals.

84 How can I lose weight when I have to eat on the run?

Plan ahead for good food choices and make use of every opportunity. It's easier to eat vegetables with ready-to-eat produce options, such as pre-washed bagged salad greens and peeled baby carrots. You may save time and money by bringing to work a low-calorie frozen entrée to pop into the microwave, or raw vegetables and fruit from home. You can build more physical activity into each day by taking a five-minute break to walk around.

As you go through your day, watch for opportunities to walk more. Use a pedometer and add a few extra steps each day. Many people gain weight because time for eating a balanced diet and being physically active are a lower priority than work or other activities. Nothing is more important than your health, exercising, and eating right. Get your priorities straight, and you can create time to take care of yourself.

To avoid confusion and indecision, set clear goals to help keep yourself organized. For example, eat an apple a day. Take the stairs. Have a salad for dinner. Make a shopping list. Cook dinner.

85 How can I lose weight and keep eating foods I like?

You do not need to give up all the foods you like. It's portion size that is important. Some foods are higher in fat content than other foods. If you cut down or cut out high-fat foods altogether, you can lose significant amounts of weight. To find the fat and caloric content of the foods you eat, check your local library, bookstore, or pharmacy for paperback books that list this information. See how much fat is in your favorite foods. Eliminating even one high-fat food that you eat often will result in weight loss. Remember that exercise makes it even easier to lose weight.

86 Does drinking water help me lose weight?

Yes, it can. Water contains no calories, and it helps you feel full. A growing number of weight- and health-conscious people have increased their daily water intake by carrying a bottle of water with them wherever they go.

Unfortunately, many people drink too many soft drinks instead of water. The obesity epidemic in our country is linked to the popularity of drinking bigger sizes of sugar-rich sports drinks and soft drinks. If you drink these instead of water, you should know that a 20-ounce soft drink contains 300–400 calories and 15–20 teaspoons of sugar. That is 12–15 calories per ounce. Fruit juices contain 12 calories per ounce, and sports drinks contain 6–10 calories per ounce. These calorie levels make water a very attractive option, indeed. If you are not a fan of water, consider seltzer (without added sugar). Diet soft drinks are another option, but for health and variety, drink water, too.

87 Won't skipping meals help me cut back on calories and lose weight?

No. Eating all your calories in one or two big meals can send your blood-sugar levels sky-high. Eating smaller meals more often keeps the amount of carbohydrates entering your system small and consistent, so your glucose level stays within your target range. This can keep your weight under control, and you'll need less insulin.

When to eat depends on many factors, particularly on the type of diabetes medication you use. If you take insulin or insulin-releasing drugs (sulfonylureas, meglitinides), skipping meals can result in dangerous hypoglycemia, and can make you hungrier, moody, and unable to focus. This may lead to overeating later in the day. Breakfast-skippers are particularly at risk for grabbing sugary, high-fat foods later in the day. Always eat within a few hours of getting up.

Your metabolism slows down when you do not eat. Eating regularly keeps your energy level high and helps your body burn calories. Eating more often doesn't mean that you eat more calories. See a registered dietitian (RD) to learn how to spread your calories throughout the day. You may find that three meals and three snacks work well for you!

88 How can I lose weight when I hardly eat anything now?

If you are not exercising, you will be surprised at the difference a daily 30-minute walk can make in both weight loss and blood-sugar control. Walking burns calories and lowers blood sugar. If exercise becomes a daily habit, you'll need to adjust the amount of insulin you take and the food you eat.

Another way to lose weight may be as simple as reducing the food you eat by one slice of bread per day. One slice of bread contains 80-100 calories, and 30 slices of bread (the amount eaten in one month) is equal to approximately one pound of body weight. Therefore, if you omit one of your usual slices of bread per day for one year, you may possibly lose up to 12 pounds!

Keep a journal of the foods you eat for 3-5 days. Also record when you eat and the emotion or situation that preceded eating. Most people are surprised to find that they eat more than they realize, or that certain situations always trigger overeating. Keeping a food diary and learning from it will help you lose weight.

89 Will a very low-calorie diet work for me?

These diets are for people with type 2 diabetes who are extremely obese and at immediate risk for serious health problems. Weight loss on a very low-calorie diet (VLCD) is rapid, and blood-sugar levels fall within a few days of beginning this restrictive way of eating. VLCDs are not for people with type 1 diabetes, because of the risk of hypoglycemia. A person with diabetes and kidney disease should not try VLCDs because of the high-protein content of the diet.

Most VLCDs are based on drinking a meal-replacement beverage or eating very lean meat. These diets are high in protein to prevent muscle tissue from wasting away and are supplemented with vitamins and minerals because so little food is eaten. Because of the side effects, VLCDs should only be used under the supervision of a physician who specializes in the care of people with diabetes and obesity.

Unfortunately, a VLCD can be expensive, and most people regain all the weight they lost within five years. It might jump-start a weight-loss effort, but for truly permanent weight-loss, you must make lasting changes in your lifestyle.

90 How can I determine my ideal body weight?

There is actually a range of body weights associated with good health. For example, a 5'5" man or woman should weigh between 114 and 150 pounds. Variables include your age, gender, body shape, and location of body fat. Talk to your health-care providers about the best weight for you.

People who are apple-shaped, who put on fat around the upper body, waist, and abdomen, tend to have more health problems than those who are pear-shaped and put on fat on the lower body, hips, and thighs. Health problems associated with apple shapes include insulin resistance, higher blood cholesterol, a tendency toward heart and blood-vessel disease, and high blood pressure.

To determine your body shape (waist-to-hip ratio):

- Measure around your waist, or one inch above your navel.
- Measure your hips at the biggest point.
- Divide your waist measurement by your hip measurement.

For a woman, a ratio greater than 0.8 is an apple shape; a ratio of less than 0.8 is a pear. For a man, a ratio greater than 1.0 is an apple, and a ratio of less than 1.0 is a pear.

91 What is BMI and why is it important?

Body mass index, or BMI, combines your weight and height into one number. BMI applies to both men and women and is related to total body fat. People whose BMI is more than 25 face an increased risk for type 2 diabetes, high blood pressure, lipid disorders, cardiovascular disease, gallbladder disease, osteoarthritis, sleep apnea, respiratory problems, and cancer. To find your BMI:

- Multiply your weight in pounds by 705.
- Divide your answer by your height in inches.
- Divide this answer by your height again.

For example, a 5'6" 185-pound individual has a BMI of about 30.

Recent guidelines define overweight as a BMI of 25-29.9, and obesity as a BMI of 30 and above. Keep in mind that the BMI is only a guideline. A very muscular, active person could have a high BMI without health risks. On the other hand, a couch potato may have a lower BMI, yet have too much body fat. If you are overweight or obese, the good news is that losing just 7 to 10% of your body weight will bring significant improvements in your health and diabetes control.

92 Why do I gain weight as I get older?

Unfortunately, most people do gain weight as they age. There are several reasons. As you get older, you tend to prefer less strenuous exercise. For example, many people in their 20s and 30s jog, play tennis, work out at health clubs, etc. In later years, they may prefer golf, bowling, and watching television. As your activities change, you burn fewer calories. If you're still eating the same amount of food that you always have, weight gain will follow.

In addition, recent studies have suggested that older people are actually more efficient at storing food as fat. This means that more exercise is needed to burn the same amount of food eaten. You should gradually decrease the amount of food that you eat as you get older to keep your body weight normal. In general, the leaner you are, the longer you will live.

93 Does insulin resistance lead to weight gain?

Scientific evidence suggests the opposite: that being overweight causes insulin resistance. Most Americans are gaining weight instead of losing it because we are eating more total calories (100–300 extra calories per day) and exercising less. Many overweight adults eat too many calories from carbohydrate-rich foods as they try to cut back on fatty foods. Eating too many carbohydrates if you are insulin resistant will raise blood-sugar levels as well as contribute extra calories. To lose weight successfully and reduce insulin resistance, reduce your calories by decreasing carbohydrates and fats in your diet. Any diet with fewer calories than you usually eat will help you lose weight and reduce insulin resistance. The key is to find a pattern of eating that healthily balances all the food groups and is lower in calories than your usual diet.

94 I binge-eat under stress. How can I avoid overeating the next time I feel pressured?

Learn the difference between hunger and appetite. Hunger is a physical sensation that alerts you when your body needs food. Appetite comes from the mind and is triggered by sensation and emotion. The following are several ways to deal with the urge to "feed your feelings" or binge:

* Identify the situations that cause you to overeat. Keep a diary of how much you eat, when you eat, and what the triggers are.
* Establish regular eating patterns. Skipping meals or not eating enough leads to overeating.
* Limit foods that tempt you. If it's chocolate, don't bring full-sized candy bars into the house; a fun-sized bar may satisfy the craving.
* Change the ways you cope with stress. When hungry, consider doing the following instead:

  ○ Exercise. Being active (walking, biking) is good for your mind and your body.
  ○ Talk with a supportive friend or family member.
  ○ Enjoy a warm bath or long shower.
  ○ Take good care of yourself. Listen to music you enjoy, go to a movie, or get a massage.

Stress can affect your blood sugar in several ways. Discuss your reactions to stress with your health-care team.

95 How can I say no to friends who push food?

It's hard to say no to friends and family. Mothers often express their love for their families by cooking favorite meals. Socializing with friends and family often takes place around food. Food has many emotional meanings, so people can be offended when you reject the food they offer.

Talking to others about why managing your weight is important to you is the first step in helping them understand. Sometimes you can suggest trying a healthier food, or take a small piece of the item offered. Serious food pushers may not respond to more subtle approaches. When a polite "No, thank you" won't work, you may need to say, "I feel that I have trouble controlling my weight and my health when I eat with you. Please support me in my decision to avoid eating seconds (or whatever you have decided to do)." If you can get them on your side, you'll both win.

96 Why would my spouse try to sabotage my diet?

If family members and friends try to lure you away from your diet or criticize your weight-loss efforts, you can feel sabotaged. Let them know that you feel discouraged by their words or actions. Discuss what they can do to truly support your efforts.

Think about your goals and how your weight loss may change your relationships. Sometimes the saboteur enjoys eating and wants you to be a partner in the fun of feasting. State your goals clearly to show that you are seriously trying to change the way you eat. It may help to consider what their goals are for you. Sometime friends and family may want your success, but feel imposed upon if you request that they keep tempting foods out of the house. You may need to negotiate an acceptable plan.

If your family and friends are aware of their ambivalent feelings about your weight loss, you may be able to discuss how they view the pros and cons. But many times the people sabotaging your efforts are unaware of their feelings. If you have difficulty talking about this together, you might discuss the problem with a professional counselor or your health-care provider.

97 What does exercise do for me?

The benefits of exercise are many, and they include:

- Strong muscles
- Increased energy
- One-pound weight loss for every 3,500 calories burned
- Improved mobility and range of joint motion
- Enhanced quality of life and independence
- A better mental attitude and self-image
- Improved blood-sugar control
- Reduced risk of heart attack and stroke
- Improved cholesterol and lipids
- Improved blood pressure
- Improved blood flow (reduced chances of conditions such as phlebitis)
- Improved appetite
- Improved enjoyment of sex
- Improved ability to play with your children or grandchildren
- Respect from your children

Exercise keeps you young and healthy. Are there any good reasons *not* to exercise?

98 How do I know I'm healthy enough to exercise?

Before starting an exercise program, you should have a health evaluation, especially if you:

- Are over 35 years old
- Have had type 2 diabetes for more than 10 years or type 1 diabetes for more than 15 years
- Have diabetes-related eye or kidney problems (retinopathy or nephropathy)
- Have poor circulation in your legs
- Have neuropathy preventing an increase in heart rate with exercise
- Have high blood pressure
- Smoke

Your doctor can help you determine whether you have any conditions that would limit the way you exercise. If you have eye problems, don't do any jumping or jarring exercise, or lift heavy weights. If you have lost feeling in your feet, be careful not to injure them—swimming may be preferable to jogging. An exercise tolerance test is important if you have heart disease.

99   I've had type 2 diabetes for 20 years and want to start exercising. What do I need to know?

Start slowly with walking or a yoga or tai chi class. Here are some basic tips:

- Before any physical activity, warm up your bones, joints, and muscles for 5-10 minutes by swinging your arms and marching, for example.
- After you are warmed up, gently stretch for another 5-10 minutes. Never stretch cold muscles. Don't bounce.
- While exercising, move quickly enough to get your heart and lungs working.
- Protect your feet. Wear good walking or running shoes with cushioned innersoles that fit well. Wear socks made of a fabric that keeps your feet dry.
- Inspect your feet regularly for blisters or injury.
- Drink water before, during, and after exercise.
- Lift some light weights. Even one-pound cans of soup can build muscle—and muscle burns calories even when you are at rest! Don't carry weights while you're walking because that can damage your wrist, elbow, and shoulder joints. Never wear ankle weights while walking!
- Keep your knees slightly bent, not locked.
- After exercise, spend 5-10 minutes cooling down, moving slower and slower. Try some yoga stretches.

100 Do I need a snack when I exercise?

If you take insulin or oral diabetes medication, it will depend on your blood-sugar level. Check your levels before and after exercise and during long, hard exercise. If your blood sugar is more than 250 mg/dl, do not exercise until it's under control. The following guidelines help maintain blood-sugar levels while exercising:

30 minutes of low-intensity exercise (walking): If your blood sugar is less than 100 mg/dl before exercise, eat a snack with 15 grams of carbohydrates.

30-60 minutes of moderate-intensity exercise (tennis, swimming, jogging): If your blood sugar is less than 100 mg/dl before exercise, have a snack with 25-50 grams of carbohydrates. If your blood sugar is 100-180 mg/dl, eat 10-15 grams of carbohydrates.

1-2 hours of strenuous-intensity exercise (basketball, skiing, shoveling snow): If your blood sugar is less than 100 mg/dl before exercise, eat a snack with about 50 grams of carbohydrates. If your blood sugar is 100-180 mg/dl, eat a snack with 25-50 grams of carbohydrates. If your blood sugar is 180-250 mg/dl, have a snack with 10-15 grams of carbohydrates. At this intense level of exercise, always monitor your blood sugar carefully.

101 Does exercise raise or lower my blood sugar?

This depends on how much insulin is in your blood. Muscles use glucose, so your blood-sugar level drops during exercise. This level will go even lower if you have a lot of insulin in your blood. However, you need some insulin circulating in your blood or, in response to exercise, your liver will make more glucose, causing your blood-sugar level to rise.

Check your blood sugar before you exercise. If it's low, you can drink a sugar-containing beverage. If it's high, you can take a small dose of regular (or lispro) insulin. If it is higher than 300 mg/dl, we recommend that you delay exercise until the insulin you have taken lowers your glucose to less than 250 mg/dl. The more intensely you exercise, the more difficult it is to predict whether your blood sugar will increase or decrease. If you exercise for a long time, recheck your blood sugar halfway through. With experience, you will learn to predict how your exercise will affect your blood-sugar levels. You may notice a blood-sugar lowering effect for as long as 24 hours after heavy exercise.

102 How do I get the regular exercise that I need to improve my blood sugar?

Walk. Many people are surprised to learn that walking is excellent exercise; we recommend it for everyone. You burn approximately 200 calories in a one-hour walk. This means you will lose one pound every three weeks from one hour of walking five days a week (providing that you don't increase the amount of food you eat). Walk to the shopping center, the supermarket, or the corner drugstore instead of driving. Walking is easy on the muscles and joints, and rarely causes low blood sugar. Exercise may make your body more sensitive to insulin, so it can help you achieve a normal body weight and a normal blood-sugar level. Start walking today!

103 I have arthritis in my hips. Can you recommend exercises other than walking?

Many people with arthritic pain in their hips or knees cannot walk the 30–60 minutes that are recommended to improve blood-sugar control. You can do armchair aerobics and stretches while sitting. Water aerobics in a swimming pool is another activity that does not put stress on your joints. If you can do them, gentle "standing" exercises, such as tai chi or chi kung, can give you a no-impact workout. All exercise routines should include a 10-minute warm-up period, 10–30 minutes of exercise, and a 10-minute cooldown period. The exercise must be intense enough to raise your heart rate but not so intense that you can't speak. You may break out in a light sweat if you're not in a pool.

Weight loss is not the only benefit of exercising. Exercise also increases insulin sensitivity, improves blood flow to the heart and muscles, and helps improve blood-sugar control. As with all exercise programs, you should consult your health-care team for recommendations about the activity that is right for you. Don't let your arthritis prevent you from exercising.

104 **What kind of exercise burns enough calories to lose weight?**

To lose a pound of body weight you need to burn 3,500 calories—not all at once, but over several days. Most people lose weight by getting more exercise each day and cutting back their food by about 500 calories a day.

The more frequently and more intensely you exercise, the more calories you burn. Exercise includes everyday activities, such as vacuuming and gardening. If you are moderately active every day, you will burn about 150 calories, or about 1,000 calories a week. With exercise alone and no diet changes, you would lose one pound over three or four weeks. A combination of exercise and chores gives you variety.

Calorie-Burning Activities Per Body Weight

Activity (30 Minutes)	Body Weight	
	120 lbs	170 lbs
Aerobic dance	165 Calories	230 Calories
Bicycling	110	155
Bowling	85	115
Gardening	140	195
Golf (walking)	125	175
Hiking	165	230
Housework	70	95

Activity (30 Minutes)	Body Weight	
	120 lbs	170 lbs
Mowing lawn	150	215
Swimming leisurely	165	230
Tennis	195	270
Walking briskly	110	155

MEDICATIONS

105 What is the best medication to treat diabetes?

There are many factors that help you and your doctor decide which is the best medication for you. People with type 2 diabetes who are overweight often release adequate amounts of insulin from their pancreas, but their muscle and fat cells are unable to respond normally, and their liver manufactures large amounts of excess glucose. For these people, metformin may be a good choice for initial therapy because it is very effective and doesn't cause weight gain.

Patients who have insufficient amounts of insulin may respond better to sulfonylureas. Other people may have problems with their blood sugar rising immediately following meals. Alpha-glucosidase inhibitors or meglitinides may be good choices for these people. These factors, along with your current blood-sugar levels and the potency, or strength, of the different medications, help you and your doctor select the most appropriate medication for you. While there may be several possible medications to control your blood sugar, other factors, such as the cost of the medication, the times per day you have to take it, pre-existing health problems (called "contraindications"), and possible side effects, also help determine which medication is best for you.

106 Is there a best time of day to take my medication?

This depends on how many times daily you are supposed to take it. If you take once-daily medications with the same meal each day, you're less likely to forget to take them. It's best to take twice-daily medications with breakfast and your evening meal. Repaglinide (Prandin), nateglinide (Starlix), acarbose (Precose), and miglitol (Glyset) should generally be taken three times daily with meals. Metformin should be taken with meals, whether taken two or three times daily for the immediate-release form, or once daily with your evening meal for the extended-release form.

107 How can I remember to take my diabetes pills to prevent high blood sugar?

The best way to remember to take medication is to always take it at the same time of day and in the same location, such as in the bathroom or at the breakfast table. To further reduce the chance of forgetting to take your medication, use a labeled pill box or pill organizer. These inexpensive boxes are available at drugstores. Dispense your daily medications in the pill box for a week at a time so you can easily keep track of whether you have taken all your pills. The more medications you take, and the more complicated your pill-taking schedule is, the more likely you are to make mistakes. The danger of not taking your diabetes medication is dangerously high blood-sugar levels.

108 What should I do if I forget to take my diabetes pills?

If you forget to take your oral diabetes medication, follow these general guidelines: If you are within three hours of the missed dose and you normally take pills twice a day, go ahead and take your medication. If more than three hours have passed, wait for your next scheduled dose. If you are on a long-acting medication that you take once a day, take your medication if you are within 12 hours of the missed dose. Otherwise, wait until the next scheduled time to resume taking your medication.

This plan is appropriate for oral medications in the classes of sulfonylureas, thiazolidinediones, and biguanides. For medications such as acarbose or repaglinide, wait until your next meal to take them.

109 If I forget to take my medications, should I take two pills for the next dose?

As a general rule, you can take a missed dose of any oral medication as soon as you remember it. However, if you forget to take a dose and it is almost time for your next scheduled dose, skip the missed dose and go back to your regular dosing schedule. *Do not* take a double dose.

There are some exceptions to this rule when taking certain diabetes medications. If you miss a dose of repaglinide (Prandin) or nateglinide (Starlix), taking the dose between meals could result in low blood-sugar reactions. Therefore, you should not take a missed dose of repaglinide or nateglinide between scheduled mealtimes. These medications are to be taken at mealtime only. If you miss a dose of acarbose (Precose) or miglitol (Glyset), you should resume your usual regimen at the next scheduled meal, since their action relies on slowing the absorption of high-starch foods.

110 Should I take my medication on an empty stomach or with food?

Generally most of the medications used to treat type 2 diabetes can be taken on a full or empty stomach. However, there are some exceptions:

- Acarbose (Precose) should be taken with the first bite of a meal for maximum benefit.
- Metformin should be taken with meals to minimize stomach upset.
- Replaglinide (Prandin) and nateglinide (Starlix) should be taken within 30 minutes of a meal for maximum benefit and to avoid low blood sugar.

111 My doctor wants me to take insulin, but I would rather take pills for my diabetes. What do you suggest?

If you have type 1 diabetes, pills will not work for you. You will have to take insulin injections. However, if you have type 2 diabetes, then you may respond to pills. Many doctors try pills in patients with type 2 diabetes, because pills are easier to take and have other advantages. Tell your doctor that you would like to try the pills, and if they don't work, then you're willing to take insulin injections. There is not an absolute blood test to predict how you will respond to pills. The only way to know is to try them for several weeks. Beginning to exercise or increasing your level of physical activity will help you gain better glucose control with diabetes pills.

If you have type 2 diabetes and are taking insulin, talk to your doctor. Many medications, such as metformin, pioglitazone, repaglinide, glyburide, and others, have permitted some people with diabetes to switch to pills and stop their injections. Many new diabetes medications are currently being tested, so stay in touch with your diabetes health-care team.

112 My doctor recently switched me from taking two different medications for my diabetes to insulin therapy. Does this mean my diabetes is getting worse?

Not necessarily, but it may be changing. In the early phases of type 2 diabetes, the pancreas has a greater ability to make insulin than in the later stages. Therefore, medications that stimulate the pancreas to make more insulin work better in people who have had diabetes for fewer than 10-15 years. As years go by, insulin levels decline and it becomes necessary to supplement the insulin made by the pancreas with insulin injections.

Other possible explanations for rising blood-sugar levels include weight gain, a decline in your activity or exercise level, a change in your eating habits, taking your medication irregularly, illness, infection, or emotional stress. Depending on your glucose level and other medical conditions, insulin may be needed, either temporarily or permanently.

113 I sometimes feel shaky, nervous, and sweaty. Is this a side effect of my diabetes medication?

Possibly, especially if you are taking any medications in the sulfonylurea class, repaglinide (Prandin), nateglinide (Starlix), or insulin. These symptoms are typical warning signs that your blood sugar is dropping below a normal level and you are experiencing hypoglycemia. Because your brain needs a certain concentration of glucose in your bloodstream to function, these symptoms generally occur when blood-sugar values fall below 70 mg/dl. However, the exact concentration at which these warning symptoms occur varies from person to person.

The causes of these symptoms may include taking too high a dose or too many medications, skipping a meal, sustained exercise, a drug interaction of your diabetes medication and another medication, or a change in your kidney or liver function (or other endocrine dysfunction, major weight loss, and/or other new comorbid conditions). It's very important to recognize these symptoms and figure out the cause so you can appropriately treat your hypoglycemia and prevent it next time. If you have frequent hypoglycemia, notify your health-care provider, since you may need your medication dose reduced.

114 My doctor warned me that I am taking the highest possible dose of glimepiride and that I may need to inject insulin in the future. I am extremely afraid of needles. Is there any way I can avoid insulin therapy?

It depends. There may be other treatment options you can request to delay the need for insulin therapy. Studies show that when you add a medication to your plan that lowers your blood sugar in a different way than your current medications, you might be able to lower your blood sugar further. Taking a combination of medications and faithfully following your meal plan and exercise program may help delay the need for insulin therapy.

Over time, however, the pancreas of many people with type 2 diabetes stops producing insulin. At this point, they must inject insulin to control their blood-sugar levels. Some people inject a small dose of insulin at bedtime while continuing to take their medication(s) during the day. While it's normal to fear needles, it may surprise you that the injections are relatively painless. The insulin injection goes into the fat layer beneath your skin where there are fewer nerve endings, using very short and thin, fine-gauge needles. Proper training on injection techniques will decrease your anxiety and discomfort, and will help you adapt to insulin therapy quite easily.

115 I have controlled my diabetes with diet, but my doctor recently prescribed a medication. Do I still need to follow my diet?

Absolutely. The very first step in treating type 2 diabetes is dietary improvement combined with exercise to achieve and maintain your desired body weight and lower your blood-sugar levels. Medications are added to diet and exercise therapy when blood-sugar levels exceed your recommended goals. Although some patients can control their blood sugar and avoid taking medication by following their meal plans and getting regular exercise, most eventually require the help of medications as well. Typically, a single medication is added to diet and exercise, using the smallest dose that will help you achieve the desired blood-sugar range.

All medications (including insulin) work best when you follow dietary guidelines designed by a registered dietitian (RD). By following your meal plan, you may be able to control your diabetes with low doses of a single medication. It is worthwhile to keep your medication plan as simple as you can for as long as possible.

116 Should I expect my blood sugars to level off after I start a new diabetes medicine?

Yes. Blood sugars initially fall in response to the medicine. But if your blood sugar has been high for some time, your pancreas can't immediately readjust because your body has been using insulin poorly. When you interrupt the cycle and spend more time in the normal blood-sugar range, you begin to increase your body's ability to stay there. After several weeks of improved control, many patients find that they need less insulin or oral medication to maintain appropriate blood-sugar levels. It may take more medication initially to begin reducing your blood sugars, but the dosage may decrease as your overall diabetes control improves.

Some patients with type 2 diabetes who take a diabetes medication and who also start exercising and eating better find that, after a while, they can stop their medication as long as they continue the other activities. Talk to your health-care team before stopping any medication. If you get the go-ahead, monitor your blood sugars while continuing your diet and exercise program. However, at the first sign that your blood-sugar levels are increasing, contact your health-care team.

117 During the holidays, when I know I will eat more, can I increase the amount of medication I take to keep my blood sugar under control?

For insulin therapy, it's possible to adjust the amount of insulin to match the carbohydrate portion, but determining how to adjust an oral medication in a similar manner is very difficult. Increasing the dose of your oral diabetes medication during the holidays may result in a low blood-sugar reaction. A better idea is to try to stick to your meal plan as much as possible and increase the frequency of your blood-sugar testing to detect any significant elevations in your blood-sugar levels.

118 What medications are available to treat type 2 diabetes?

Along with insulin, there are six classes of medications available to treat type 2 diabetes. The table below describes the medications in each class. Generally, medications in the same class are not used together because they have the same effect.

Classes of Diabetes Medications

Medication Class	Generic Name *Available Generically	Brand Name
alpha-Glucosidase Inhibitors	Acarbose	Precose
	Miglitol	Glyset
Biguanides	Metformin*	Glucophage
	Metformin* *(long-acting)*	Glucophage XR, Glumetza, others
	Metformin *(liquid)*	Riomet
DPP-4 Inhibitors	Sitagliptin	Januvia
Meglitinides *(Can cause low blood sugar, but risk is lower than with sulfonylureas.)*	Nateglinide	Starlix
	Repaglinide	Prandin
Thiazolidinediones *(TZDs)*	Pioglitazone	Actos
	Rosiglitazone	Avandia

Medication Class	Generic Name *Available Generically	Brand Name
Sulfonylureas (*These drugs can cause low blood sugar.*)	Glimepiride*	Amaryl
	Glipizide*	Glucotrol
	Glipizide* (*long-acting*)	Glucotrol XL
	Glyburide*	DiaBeta, Micronase
	Glyburide* (*micronized*)	Glynase PresTab
	Chlorpropamide*	Diabinese
	Tolazamide*	generic only
	Tolbutamide*	generic only
Combination Pills	Metformin Glyburide*	Glucovance
	Metformin Rosiglitazone	Avandamet
	Metformin Glipizide*	Metaglip
	Metformin Pioglitazone	Actoplus Met
	Metformin Sitagliptin	Janumet
	Pioglitazone Glimepiride	Duetact
	Rosiglitazone Metformin	Avandaryl

119 How do the medications listed in Tip 118 work to lower my blood sugar?

All of these medications work differently. The chart below describes their main site of action in the body and the way in which they lower blood sugar.

How Classes of Diabetes Medications Work

Medication Class	Site of Action	Action
alpha-Glucosidase inhibitors (e.g., acarbose, miglitol)	Digestive system	Slows the breakdown of starches to glucose. Slows the entry of glucose into the bloodstream after a meal.
Biguanides (e.g., metformin)	Liver	Decreases glucose production by the liver.
Meglitinides (e.g., repaglinide, nateglinide)	Pancreas	Stimulates insulin release by the pancreas in response to a meal.
Sulfonylureas	Pancreas	Stimulates insulin release by the pancreas.
Thiazolidinediones (e.g., pioglitazone, rosiglitazone)	Muscle	Enhances glucose uptake by the muscle. Improves the body's sensitivity to insulin

120 **Do all medications used to treat type 2 diabetes work equally well?**

No. Type 2 medications differ in the way they work and have different potencies, or strengths, for lowering your blood sugar. As a general rule, the sulfonylureas, repaglinide, and biguanides are more potent in lowering blood sugar than are the thiazolidinediones or alpha-glucosidase inhibitors when used as single agents. The chart below shows how effectively various medications lower glucose levels.

Blood-Sugar Effectiveness of Diabetes Medications

Medication Class	Decreases Fasting Blood Sugar by:*	Decreases A1C by:*
alpha-Glucosidase Inhibitors (e.g., acarbose)	10–20 mg/dl	0.5–1.0%
Biguanides (e.g., metformin)	50–70 mg/dl	1.5–1.7%
Meglitinides (eg., repaglinide)	60–70 mg/dl	1.5–1.7%
Meglitinides (eg., nateglinide)	60–70 mg/dl	1.5–1.7%
Sulfonylureas	50–70 mg/dl	1.5–1.7%
Thiazolidinediones (e.g., pioglitazone, rosiglitazone)	40 mg/dl	0.8–1.5%

* *Each person responds differently.*

121 Do diabetes pills contain insulin?

No. These medications help your pancreas release more insulin or help your own body's insulin work better to lower your blood sugar. Therefore, you must have a pancreas that makes and releases insulin for these medications to work (the exceptions are metformin, pioglitazone, or rosiglitazone, which work well with injected insulin). Over time, some people with type 2 diabetes no longer are able to produce any insulin on their own and must be treated with insulin injections.

122 **I have many friends and relatives with type 2 diabetes and not one of us is being treated with the same medication. Why are there so many differences in the way we are treated?**

With type 1 diabetes, the treatment is very straightforward. Because your pancreas no longer produces insulin, you must inject insulin. The treatment of type 2 diabetes is not as simple, because this type of diabetes is caused by many factors: a pancreas that does not produce enough insulin, a liver that makes too much glucose, or muscle cells that are not able to take in the glucose and use it for energy. Different medications are now available that treat these different causes of diabetes. Additionally, some treatments may work through a mechanism that is not directly a contributory cause of the diabetes (for example, SGLT-2 inhibitors). Sometimes these medications are used in combination with each other or with insulin. The goal is to get enough insulin in your body—whether it comes from your pancreas with the help of medications, or is injected—to move glucose into your cells to use as energy.

123 Which type 2 medication should I use?

You and your health-care provider must discuss this. There are several different classes of medicine that treat diabetes, and the one you should use depends on dosing requirements, side effects, hypoglycemia risk, cost, and—most importantly—whether it enables you to meet your target blood-sugar goals. If you are unable to meet your target goals with only one agent, your health provider may place you on two or more drugs to try to control your diabetes.

124 I have had type 2 diabetes for years and started taking insulin before many new oral medications were available. Is it possible I could control my blood sugar using an oral and/ or non-insulin injectable medication or a combination of medications?

Yes. Some diabetes specialists have successfully converted people with type 2 diabetes from insulin-only therapies to a combination of oral medications. Generally, these people were switched from medications to insulin during a time when the only oral medications available to treat diabetes were sulfonylureas. Even though there were several different medications within this group, they all had a similar chemical structure and acted in the same way. When people no longer responded to these medications over time, the only other option was insulin.

Now there are several new medications that lower blood sugar in different ways. In general, you have the best chance of responding to a combination of oral medications if your total daily insulin requirement is less than 40 units daily, your current plasma glucose values are within the target range recommended by the ADA (between 90 and 130 mg/dl), and you've had diabetes for fewer than 15 years.

125 Are there any useful herbal remedies for diabetes?

We don't know. Diet and herbal remedies were the only treatments available for most of the 2,000 years since diabetes was first described. Health-food stores carry dozens of products designed for people with diabetes, ranging from blueberry leaf and wild cherry bark to preparations such as Hysugar and Losugar. Few of these products have been tested or proven to be safe and effective. Because herbal remedies are classified as food supplements, they are not regulated by the Food and Drug Administration (FDA). Moreover, none of these products alone result in adequate blood-sugar control in most people with diabetes.

You should discuss any anti-diabetes health-food products with your health-care team. You may find that they are somewhat skeptical, but they will probably not object to using these products in moderation if you demonstrate good diabetes control and do what's necessary to stay healthy.

126 Are there any health benefits to fish oil?

Possibly. People with diabetes typically have elevated levels of fatty particles in their blood known as triglycerides. High triglyceride levels are one of the reasons that people with diabetes have an increased risk for heart disease. Oils from a variety of fish, such as sardines, may lower blood triglyceride concentrations in patients with diabetes, according to 26 separate studies. Specifically, 2-5 teaspoons of fish oil were shown to reduce triglyceride levels by an average of 30-50%.

Unfortunately, the fish oil slightly raised the levels of LDL cholesterol, another fatty particle that is connected to heart disease. Also, blood-sugar levels showed a slight increase by the daily use of fish oil. For now, you might consider replacing red meat in your diet with fish several times a week. If you have high triglyceride levels, ask your doctor about the possibility of including a daily dose of fish oil.

127 Do people with diabetes have special needs for vitamins? If so, which ones should I take?

People with diabetes do have special needs for vitamins and minerals. When your blood-sugar levels are high, glucose spills into your urine, leading to an increase in urination. This may lead to excessive losses of magnesium, zinc, and water-soluble vitamins such as Vitamin C. Those taking Metformin may be at an increased risk for Vitamin B12 deficiency. Also, many people with diabetes are on weight-reduction plans and may not be eating a well-balanced diet. Nonprescription multivitamin and mineral products can help replace these possible deficits, but be sure to discuss any additional supplementation with your physician. Try to eat a well-balanced, healthy diet and take an inexpensive, all-purpose multivitamin and mineral product daily.

128 Should I take an aspirin daily if I have diabetes?

Probably. Diabetes increases your risk of dying from complications of heart and cardiovascular disease. In November 1997, the ADA concluded that low-dose aspirin therapy should be prescribed, not only for patients with diabetes who have had heart attacks, but also for patients with diabetes who are at a high risk for future heart and artery disease. This includes both men and women. People with diabetes may be at a greater risk because their platelets (parts of cells circulating in the blood that clump and prevent bleeding) may clump more spontaneously than in people who do not have diabetes. Aspirin prevents this clumping and, therefore, may prevent heart attacks.

Taking aspirin, however, is not without risk. It can cause stomach and intestinal bleeding, so people with bleeding ulcers shouldn't take aspirin. However, the risk is greatly reduced if you take enteric-coated aspirin of 81–325 milligrams a day. In fact, the lower dose (81 milligrams) of enteric-coated aspirin has been shown to be just as effective as higher doses in preventing platelets from clumping. You should discuss the use of aspirin with your physician to make sure that it's safe for you.

129 **Many medications you can buy without a prescription say "consult with your physician before using if you have diabetes." Should I heed these warnings? Are there general rules for buying medications without a prescription?**

Yes. Always read the labels carefully to see whether a product contains sugar or alcohol. Look in the active and inactive ingredients sections. Use tablets or capsules when possible, since they generally contain less sugar and alcohol compared to liquid products. Avoid combination products that are designed to treat a variety of symptoms, as they tend to have hidden ingredients that could be harmful.

Some over-the-counter products may have harmful side effects that can increase or decrease your blood sugar and worsen diabetic complications, such as nerve or kidney disease. Some have a negative effect on other conditions, such as high blood pressure or high blood lipids. Therefore, it is very important to read labels and heed any warnings regarding diabetes, high blood pressure, or heart disease. If such warnings are present, ask your physician or pharmacist if the product is safe for you to take.

130 Should I tell my physician if I am taking any medications I purchased without a prescription?

Yes. Always tell your physician, pharmacist, and other health-care providers about any over-the-counter products you take. Like all medications, these products can cause harmful side effects, even though you don't need a prescription for them. Your physician and pharmacist can check the product to see if it negatively interacts with any medications you are currently taking, or if it could make any of your current medical conditions worse. When telling your physician or pharmacist which over-the-counter medications you are taking, be sure to include dietary supplements, such as vitamins and minerals, and herbal products, including herbal teas.

131 Will the medication I am taking for depression affect my blood sugar?

Probably not. Depression is more common in patients with chronic diseases such as diabetes. Up to 40% of people with diabetes may have depression at some point in their lives. Medications for depression have no major direct impact on how your oral diabetes medications or insulin work to control your blood sugar.

On the other hand, giving adequate attention to diabetes management can seem impossible if you are depressed. While there are many ways to deal with depression, sometimes several months of treatment with medication helps you to get back to being yourself faster. A vicious cycle can develop where high blood sugars make you feel sleepy and sap you of energy to get out and exercise. But exercise would help lower your blood sugar and make you feel better physically and mentally. Dealing with depression can break the cycle and put you back on track, eating right and exercising, to help you feel better all the time.

132 Is it safe for me to use birth-control pills if I have diabetes?

Birth-control pills appear to be safe for women with diabetes, and they are certainly safer than a pregnancy for which you are unprepared. Diabetes specialists disagree about the best form of birth control for women with diabetes. Under certain circumstances, estrogen-containing birth-control pills may affect blood-sugar and blood-cholesterol levels. For this reason, some physicians do not prescribe them for women with diabetes.

Studies have shown, however, that blood-sugar levels are no different in women who take birth-control pills than in women who do not. Similarly, blood-cholesterol and lipid levels are no different in women with diabetes who use birth-control pills than in those who do not. There are other effective birth-control methods, such as a diaphragm, that do not affect blood sugar at all. Talk to your health-care team about which birth-control method will work best for you.

If you have peripheral vascular disease (blood-circulation problems), birth-control pills can increase your risk for blood clots. However, the doses of estrogen used in most birth-control pills now are much lower than doses used in the past, so this problem is more rare than it used to be.

Women who smoke or have diabetes are at an increased risk of cardiovascular events, such as stroke and clots in peripheral blood vessels. To minimize this risk, use a low-dose estrogen product, keep your blood-sugar levels under control, and do not smoke.

Women over 35 who are heavy smokers (more than 15 cigarettes a day) should not take birth-control pills due to a substantially increased risk for stroke, heart attack, and blood clots. All women should quit smoking, preferably with the help of a counseling program. At the very minimum, an alternate type of birth control is recommended.

133 Why are my blood sugars high while I am taking prednisone for my asthma?

Prednisone is used for a variety of conditions such as asthma and other lung problems. It acts like a hormone called "cortisol" that your body makes. Cortisol and prednisone both cause the body to make glucose when you're not eating, such as during the night. They can worsen diabetes control. Cortisol is a "stress hormone" because the body releases it to deal with stresses like accidents, infections, or burns. That's partly why your body takes more insulin to keep blood sugars near normal during an infection.

If you're taking prednisone and you have diabetes, you may need to take more diabetes medication. Your health-care team can help you alter your diabetes treatment, if necessary, until you can stop taking the prednisone. Prednisone's effect on your blood sugar will go away a day or two after you stop taking it.

FOOT ISSUES

134 Will I have foot problems because I have diabetes?

People with diabetes have the same foot problems that people without diabetes experience—corns, calluses, bunions, ingrown toenails, arthritis, and broken bones. However, these ordinary foot problems can be more serious in people with diabetes if they also have diabetic nerve disease or poor circulation.

People with diabetic nerve damage have no feeling in their feet, so they may not notice an injury, sores, or even high-pressure areas on their feet. They may continue to walk on an injury or high-pressure spot that would cause pain in a person without nerve damage. This continued walking might cause a wound or ulcer. Once the skin is broken, the ulcer can become infected. The blood supply carries oxygen, white blood cells that attack bacteria, and healing nutrients to wounds. It also carries any antibiotics that you take. But if you don't have enough blood supply to the foot, an ulcer can be difficult or impossible to heal. If left untreated, foot infections can lead to amputation.

135 Why is it important for me to take special care of my feet?

If you want to be active and independent all of your life—whether or not you have diabetes—you need to have healthy feet. Most people take their feet for granted, but people with diabetes can't. You are challenged by two complications of diabetes that can affect the nerves and blood vessels in the feet—diabetic nerve damage and poor circulation. These complications make it easier for you to get a foot ulcer that will not heal. Nonhealing ulcers lead to amputation, which will severely limit what you can do for yourself.

The good news is that by taking good care of your feet, you can often prevent diabetic foot complications. If you take care of your feet every day and get good medical care as soon as you even suspect you might need it, you're much more likely to avoid infections that make amputation necessary. In fact, at least 50% of amputations in people with diabetes could be prevented this way. You can protect your feet.

136 What is peripheral neuropathy?

Peripheral neuropathy is the name for damage to motor and sensory nerves. Motor and sensory nerves help you move and touch the world around you. "Peripheral" means at the edges or away from the center. In this case, the feet are farthest from the center of the body. "Neuro" means nerves and "pathy" means "a disorder of." Because the longest nerves are usually affected first, symptoms such as tingling, burning, or numbness appear first in the feet and hands. If you think of the nervous system as the electrical system in your house, then the wires to the lights and appliances are the peripheral nerves, while the fuse box and main cable are the central nervous system (the brain and spinal cord).

When motor nerves are damaged, muscles in your foot can weaken and allow the shape of the foot to change. Toes can curl up and the fat pad on the bottom of the foot can shift so that it no longer protects the skin. As a result, the bones in the foot can get very close to the skin and can cause calluses. The sensory nerve damage prevents you from feeling pain, so the callus can become an ulcer without you knowing it.

137 How does diabetes cause nerve damage?

Nobody really knows. Certainly higher than normal blood-sugar levels are part of the cause. We know that keeping your blood sugar in control can lower your chances of getting neuropathy; that people with high blood sugar are more likely to have neuropathy; and that the longer a person has diabetes, the more likely he or she is to have neuropathy.

There are several theories about how blood sugar affects nerves. One theory is that sugar coats the proteins in the nerves and that the sugar-coated proteins no longer function normally. Another theory is that high blood-sugar levels interfere with chemical events in the nerves, and possibly even damage the insulation layer of cells around the nerves. Or, it might be that high blood-sugar levels damage the tiny blood vessels that supply the nerves, cutting them off from oxygen and nutrients. Researchers are working to understand the causes of neuropathy and to find treatments to avoid the damage it causes.

138 How do I know if I have peripheral neuropathy?

If you have had diabetes for more than 10 years and you have not kept your blood-sugar levels close to near normal levels, you likely have some symptoms of nerve damage. It affects as many as 75% of all people with diabetes. Do you have muscle weakness, cramps, or feelings of numbness, tingling, pins and needles, and burning sensations in your feet and legs? Do your feet bother you more at night? Have you had any episodes of fainting or vomiting or had a change in bowel habits, bladder control, or sexual functioning? These systems can be affected by diabetic nerve damage, too.

There is not one specific test for diabetic nerve damage. Generally, if you have two or more symptoms and a positive test for loss of sensation—you cannot feel the touch of a plastic wire or a vibrating tuning fork on the bottom of your foot—you will be diagnosed as having neuropathy.

139 Does diabetes cause more than one kind of neuropathy?

Yes. Diabetic nerve damage can affect three kinds of nerves in your body: nerves you use for feeling (sensory neuropathy), nerves that go to the muscles (motor neuropathy), and nerves that control automatic body activities such as blood flow and digestion (autonomic neuropathy). With sensory nerve damage, you may not be able to feel heat and cold and may have tingling, pain, or numbness. When this occurs in your feet, you may be more likely to fall. With motor nerve damage, muscles are weakened and you are more likely to develop foot deformities such as hammertoes.

Damage to autonomic nerves can affect major systems in your body, such as the heart, stomach, or sexual organs. It can affect heart rate and blood pressure. It can cause gastroparesis and erectile dysfunction. This type of nerve damage also can interfere with the functioning of your bladder, eyes, and sweat glands, and can lead to hypoglycemia awareness (symptoms of low blood sugar).

The best way to prevent nerve damage is to keep your blood-sugar levels close to normal. Getting better blood-sugar control can help relieve symptoms of ongoing neuropathy, but you may not be able to reverse extensive damage, such as completely numb feet.

140 Are there any treatments for peripheral neuropathy?

The best treatment is to get your blood-sugar levels under control. Studies show that good blood-sugar control can help prevent any nerve damage you already have from getting worse. Take note that if you go on insulin or a sulfonylurea and improve your blood-sugar control, the pain may increase for a little while until your body gets accustomed to the lower blood-sugar levels.

Medications such as antidepressants, anticonvulsants (seizure medicine), muscle relaxants, local anesthetics (such as a lidocaine patch), anti-inflammatory drugs, vitamins, evening primrose oil, and capsaicin creams made from hot peppers have been used to treat neuropathy symptoms. Physical therapy treatments, such as stretching exercises, massage, and electrical nerve stimulation, have also been tried.

Although studies of these therapies report some improvement in painful symptoms for some patients, there is no single treatment that works for everyone. It may be difficult to get complete relief. Discuss your symptoms with your provider and try the treatment you both think might work. If that treatment doesn't help, let your provider know so you can try another.

141   What is peripheral vascular disease?

Peripheral vascular disease (PVD) is commonly called "poor circulation" and refers to blockage in the blood supply to the feet. A buildup of plaque inside the arteries that carry blood to the feet causes the arteries to thicken and harden. People without diabetes get this thickening and hardening of the arteries, too, but unfortunately these problems can happen sooner and be more severe in people with diabetes. In fact, PVD is 20 times more common in people with diabetes than in the general population.

Other things that put you at risk of developing PVD are smoking, poor nutrition, lack of exercise, high blood-fat levels (including cholesterol), and poor blood sugar control. Women and men are at equal risk, as are young and old. You can avoid or limit the risks of developing PVD by stopping smoking and controlling your blood-fat and blood-sugar levels as much as possible. See a registered dietitian (RD) for help with your meal plan and add more physical activity to your lifestyle.

142 How do I know when I have poor circulation in my feet and legs?

The hallmark of poor circulation is pain or cramping in the calf or thigh that occurs when you walk a short distance. This pain is a sign that the muscles are not getting enough oxygen. If you slow or stop and rest for a few minutes, the oxygen supply usually catches up with the demand and then you can walk a little farther before the pain reoccurs. The medical term for this condition is "intermittent claudication."

Other signs of poor circulation can be pain at rest, nonhealing ulcers, absent or weak pulses in the feet or legs, a decrease in blood pressure in the feet and legs, or a lack of hair growth on the lower legs. A blue or purplish color, especially when your feet are hanging down, and having cold feet are also signs of circulation problems.

If you think you have poor circulation to the feet, ask your provider to evaluate it. Poor circulation is caused by a blockage in the arteries supplying blood to the feet. The blockage may need to be removed or bypassed with vascular surgery. A simple treatment is to walk every day. This exercise can force the blood vessels to expand and improve the circulation in your feet and legs.

143 If my feet don't hurt, should I still check them every day?

Yes! You should examine your feet at the end of each day to look for sores, cuts, or areas where your shoe is rubbing against your foot. People with diabetes may lose pain sensation in their feet, and may develop ulcers and open sores unknowingly because they can't feel the pain. Without medical attention, sores may continue to be irritated and not heal properly. Although your health-care team should examine your feet at each visit, you need to look for any small areas of redness or bleeding.

It is essential that your shoes are comfortable and fit well, and that you always wear socks or stockings to provide padding between your feet and shoes. If your feet are difficult to fit, special shoes can be made for you. The longer a patient has diabetes, the more common foot problems are. Preventing foot sores is much easier than trying to heal them.

144   How do I know whether I have an infection?

Some signs of infection are:

- Redness
- Swelling
- Increased warmth
- Pain, tenderness, or limited motion of the affected part
- Pus or drainage from the wound

If you have one or two of these signs, have a health-care provider check your wound to determine whether you have an infection.

Other signs that an infection has spread beyond the wound are fever, chills, or an unusually high blood sugar. If you have any of these signs, see a doctor immediately or go to an emergency room if your regular health-care provider cannot see you right away.

145 Should I be concerned about a small red blister on my foot from walking in new shoes?

Yes! You may look at a small blister and think that it is nothing serious, but it can be. If the blister breaks, it can allow germs into your foot. These germs can cause not only an infection in your foot, but also in the bone. Infections in the bone are very difficult to treat and often lead to amputations.

Immediately wash your feet carefully in gentle soap and water and dry them thoroughly. Then put a small amount of antibiotic ointment on a dressing and cover the wound. Next, call your health-care team and let them know that you have a sore on your foot. Your health-care team will want to see your foot to decide whether you need to start taking antibiotics. Finally, quit wearing the shoes that caused the blister—the shoes you wear must fit your feet. A comfortable pair of shoes is one of the best investments you can make and may prevent future problems.

146 Why do my feet burn at night when I'm trying to go to sleep?

The nerves in your feet have been affected by your diabetes. "Painful neuropathy" is a term used to describe diabetic feet that are painful without an obvious cause. People with painful neuropathy usually describe a "pins and needles" sensation or a dull burning in the feet and legs that is more apparent at night when there are few other things to distract you. You may also experience frequent leg cramps.

Because painful neuropathy is difficult to cure once it is established, the best treatment is to prevent it by controlling your blood sugar. These nerve problems occur more frequently in men and in people who have had diabetes for many years, are tall, smoke, or have poor blood-sugar control.

If you already have painful neuropathy, there are treatments available that provide some relief for about 50% of people. These treatments include the use of antidepressant medicines, certain heart medications, and creams made from chili peppers (capsaicin). These creams are rubbed on the feet to desensitize them. If you do not get relief from one of these treatments, the good news is that the pain from neuropathy often lessens over time.

147 What can I do for the numbness in my feet?

This is a very serious condition. Most people go to the doctor because their foot hurts. Yours never will. You must check your feet by touching them with your hands and by looking at them every day!

Controlling your blood sugar may help prevent the numbness from getting worse. Get your shoes fitted properly, if necessary by a pedorthist, and find out whether you need special shoes to protect your feet. Before putting on your shoes, check them for foreign objects, nails, or anything that would injure your foot. Be sure your socks are not wrinkled or twisted. You may want to switch to socks without a toe seam because the seam can put pressure on your toes.

If you find the numbness is uncomfortable, discuss treatments for neuropathy with your health-care provider. Whenever you see an injury to your feet or a change in the shape of your feet, see your foot-care specialist right away. Do not wait until an infection develops!

148 Does the pain in my feet have anything to do with high blood sugar?

Probably, especially if you have had high blood sugar for many years and the pain has lasted for several months. Nerves work better when blood-sugar levels are normal rather than high. Discuss your pain with your health-care team. Some people find that the pain in their feet and legs decreases when their blood sugar is brought closer to normal. Others find it painful for bedsheets to touch their feet. If you experience this, place a hoop over the end of the bed so that the sheet is kept off of your feet. This will provide relief until you lower your blood sugars.

If the problem doesn't go away with improved blood-sugar control, then putting capsaicin cream, which is made from chili peppers, on the affected skin may help. Other therapies, especially medication, are also available, so discuss the various options with your diabetes health-care team.

149 Does my weight affect my feet?

Absolutely. The more we weigh, the more stress is transmitted through our knees, ankles, and feet. Many people with foot pain can get relief just by losing weight. Heel pain is often weight-related, and arthritis in the knees and feet is frequently worse in people who are overweight.

People who are obese have a different gait from those who are not. Their feet are placed wider than normal because their thighs hold the legs outward. This places the body weight more towards the inner part of the foot, changing completely the mechanics of walking. The result is increased stress on the tendons, ligaments, and joints of the feet.

If you have diabetic neuropathy, your weight is even more important. The stress of additional pounds on numb feet increases the likelihood of your developing ulcers and Charcot deformities (a breakdown of the arch and normal foot structure that can result in swelling, redness, and even broken bones).

If you become pregnant, your feet may change shape and size during the pregnancy and for about six months after the baby is born. Sometimes they remain permanently larger. Be aware of this and try to wear comfortable, supportive shoes, such as running shoes. High heels are not really a good idea for anyone, but especially for a pregnant woman.

150 Does a meal plan have anything to do with my feet?

Yes. You know that achieving near normal blood-sugar levels can improve your chances of not having nerve damage or circulation problems. Part of managing your blood sugar is following a meal plan, along with daily exercise and diabetes medication if you need it. In addition, we know that what you eat affects your health, including your skin, muscles, and bones. Your diet also affects your blood fats and plays an important part in circulation and peripheral vascular disease.

A meal plan that is unbalanced with too many processed foods (white flour, sugars, and fats) and too few vegetables and fruits leaves you with fewer weapons to fight against bacteria and fungus on the skin. That is why a diet for people with diabetes is the same healthy diet everyone should follow. Especially important are the vitamins and minerals that you can get from vegetables and fruits. You also want to make sure that you are getting enough calcium and magnesium for your bones. Ask for a referral to a registered dietitian (RD) if you need help designing or changing your meal plan to meet your needs and to get your blood sugar under control.

151 Will Medicare pay for my therapeutic shoes?

Medicare currently pays for therapeutic footwear when you meet certain criteria and fill out the proper forms, though coverage can change in the future. This benefit covers custom-molded shoes, extra-depth shoes, inserts, and some shoe modifications.

To take advantage of the benefit, your physician must certify that you are in a plan of diabetes care, have evidence of foot disease, and need therapeutic footwear. A podiatrist writes the prescription, and a podiatrist or pedorthist provides the shoes. You must buy the footwear from a qualified supplier and file the forms. (The forms are available from prescription shoe stores, Medicare, or a podiatrist, or your provider may help you get them.)

Usually you have to pay for the shoes, and Medicare reimburses up to 80% of the reasonable charge within limits. Ask about the charge and how much Medicare will pay when you order the shoes. Although government programs can be time-consuming, prescription footwear can be an important part of preventing foot problems.

152 Since I don't want to end up with foot problems, how do I know whether my athletic shoes are okay?

It's best to buy shoes from a store that has experienced personnel who know how to measure your feet and fit your shoes correctly. A certified pedorthist is a specialist in fitting shoes and inserts for a proper fit with no pressure points. When you get new shoes, wear them for a few hours only, and then check your feet for any red areas or sore places where the shoes might be rubbing. Even well-fitted shoes may have a seam or area that rubs on your foot. Also wear padded athletic socks to protect your feet from blisters.

Athletic shoes have become very high-tech these days and have different features for various kinds of exercise. It is a good idea to buy ones with extra cushion because this reduces the wear and tear on your joints. Look in the Yellow Pages or on the Internet for stores that specialize in athletic shoes or have a pedorthist on staff.

MISCELLANEOUS COMPLICATIONS

153 Can diabetic complications be predicted?

Sometimes. We know that certain factors, such as having consistently high blood-sugar levels, predict the development of more diabetic complications, but we cannot predict who will get which complications. Still, research studies on complications can be useful and informative. For example, one study attempted to determine the most important predictors for eye disease, kidney disease, and amputation among 2,774 patients with diabetes. This study showed that older individuals and people with less education were more likely to suffer complications.

In this same study, other factors were also important. In people with type 1 diabetes, the combination of high blood pressure and smoking were the most powerful predictors of diabetic complications. For people with type 2 diabetes, failure to seek regular

183

diabetes care was the most powerful predictor of diabetic complications. Although we can never be absolutely certain whether you will develop diabetic complications, we do know that you can minimize your risk by carefully controlling your blood sugar and blood pressure, avoiding smoking, and working with your diabetes-care team to be as healthy as you can be.

154 What kinds of eye problems are caused by diabetes?

Diabetes is the leading cause of blindness in the United States. Fortunately, many eye problems are treatable if they are identified early. One of the most serious eye problems caused by diabetes is retinopathy. In this disease, fragile blood vessels grow in the back of the eye and can bleed easily. Such bleeding can cloud the vision and lead to permanent scarring of the back of the eye (the retina).

People with diabetes also have cataracts (a permanent clouding of the lens), "floaters" that temporarily interfere with vision, and a swelling of the eye nerves that can cause permanent damage to your sight (macular edema). Abnormal function of the nerves that control the eye muscles can result in double vision. People who develop double vision should see an eye doctor as soon as possible to rule out other possible causes, such as a small stroke. Cataracts can be corrected surgically. Laser therapy helps stop retinopathy or macular edema if it is performed before there is too much damage.

A yearly eye examination by a doctor who specializes in diabetic eye disease is the best way to detect eye problems in the early stages. Also, keeping your blood sugar near normal can help reduce your risk of eye disease.

155 Does diabetes put me at risk for developing thyroid problems?

Perhaps. The thyroid gland in your neck secretes thyroid hormone. Low levels of thyroid hormone (known as "thyroid failure") are common in individuals with type 1 diabetes. Thyroid hormone gives you energy and helps maintain other organ systems in your body.

We recommend that you get a blood test for thyroid hormone once a year, particularly if you feel more tired than usual or have other symptoms, such as constipation, dry skin, and feeling cold most of the time. Treatment is easy and inexpensive. It is also very important, because when low thyroid hormone goes untreated, it can lead to many medical problems. Do not hesitate to ask your doctor periodically to check your blood thyroid hormone level. Remember that other medical problems can occur in people with diabetes that are not directly related to high blood-sugar levels.

156 Why are my fingernails thick and pulling away from the nail bed?

Your fingernails may have a fungal infection. Fungal infections of the skin, such as "athlete's foot," are more common in people with diabetes. These fungal infections can occasionally involve unusual areas of the body, such as your nails, scalp, or groin. A fungal infection in your fingernails is not a serious threat to your overall health, but it may make your nails brittle and unsightly. You can also spread the infection to other areas of your body, such as your scalp, by scratching with infected nails.

See your health-care team or a dermatologist to treat the infection. This involves taking a sample from under your nails and examining it under the microscope to confirm the diagnosis. Nail infections are difficult to cure, and you will probably require treatment with an oral drug for several months. Because these drugs may damage your liver or bone marrow, you may need to take blood tests every few weeks to monitor your blood-cell counts and your liver function. After all of this effort, you may be rewarded with a return of healthy fingernails.

157 Am I more likely to develop skin infections because I have diabetes?

You may be. People with diabetes who are over-weight or who have high blood sugars most of the time are more likely to develop skin infections than are thin people with normal blood sugars. High blood sugars can interfere with your body's natural defense systems. Once they start, some of these infections can spread rapidly, causing fever, chills, and tiredness.

It is very important that you examine your skin each day and promptly take care of any ulcers, red-ness, or skin breakdowns. Yeast infections usually occur in warm, moist areas of the body, particularly in the genital region, under breasts, and between folds of skin. Infections of the face, foot, and ear canal may be particularly serious and should be checked by your health-care team.

Many different types of treatments are avail-able for these skin problems, and you should ask for advice before applying drugstore skin creams. Good skin care is essential for good health.

158 Can diabetes cause diarrhea?

Yes. Frequent diarrhea occurs in 5–20% of people with long-standing diabetes. The possible causes include fewer digestive enzymes being released from the pancreas, overuse of magnesium-containing antacids, or too many bacteria in the upper part of the intestine where they should not normally be. Often, however, the cause is unknown, but damage to the nerves that control bowel movement is thought to be a basic cause.

See your health-care team for an evaluation. If you don't have enough digestive enzymes, a pill taken with meals may cure the problem. If the cause of your diarrhea remains unknown, other treatments may help harden your stools and decrease the number of daily bowel movements. Some of these treatments include simple over-the-counter remedies like psyllium (Metamucil) or a kaolin and pectin mixture (Kaopectate).

Other people respond to prescription drugs, such as cholesterol-binding resins (cholestyramine), antibiotics (tetracycline or erythromycin), or drugs designed to decrease movement in the bowel, such as loperamide (Lomotil). Some people get diarrhea when taking Metformin. If the maximum dose is in place, sometimes the problem may be solved by a dose reduction. Whatever the cause of your diarrhea, you deserve a careful medical review of this problem, because chances are good that some of your symptoms can be relieved.

159 Why do I sometimes leak urine?

Approximately 25% of all people with long-term diabetes have some problems with bladder function. Most of these problems result from faulty signals from the nerves that control the bladder. Some of these problems are minor, such as an inability to empty your bladder completely when you urinate, or a slow rate of urine flow. A more advanced problem is incontinence, when you accidentally leak urine. The most common cause of incontinence is an inability to tell whether your bladder is full, causing it to fill until it overflows. Men with incontinence often have an enlarged prostate gland pressing on the bladder, which can be treated with medicine or corrected by surgery. All men with diabetes over 40 should have a prostate exam every year.

If you have overflow incontinence, you may be able to manage the problem by reminding yourself to urinate on a schedule every day. You may strengthen the muscles around the bladder by doing kegel exercises (tensing and relaxing the pelvic muscles), or stopping the flow of urine several times. If you continue to have trouble, seek help from a bladder specialist (a urologist).

160 Is insulin resistance important to my diabetes? What can I do about it?

Yes, insulin resistance makes diabetes worse. We don't know why people with diabetes have insulin resistance. Physicians recommend several ways to reduce insulin resistance to make your own insulin more effective and better able to control your blood sugar. The nondrug ways to reduce insulin resistance are a low-calorie diet, weight loss, and regular and vigorous exercise. In other words, a healthy lifestyle can help you reduce insulin resistance.

Many medications have been approved by the Food and Drug Administration (FDA) for type 2 diabetes, but three drugs also reduce insulin resistance and, therefore, improve diabetes control. Metformin acts on your liver and, to a lesser extent, on your muscles to reduce insulin resistance. Pioglitazone (Actos) and rosiglitazone (Avandia) have been shown to act in the liver, muscles, and fat tissue to reduce insulin resistance. These medications are widely used in managing type 2 diabetes and are very effective. If you have type 2 diabetes, discuss with your health provider which approaches are best for you to reduce the insulin resistance in your body.

DIABETES AND PREGNANCY

161 What are the risks to my baby during my pregnancy?

Pregnancy in diabetes carries risks for both you and your baby. Babies born to mothers with diabetes have higher rates of birth defects and stillbirth. The babies can also be abnormally large, which complicates the delivery. You can avoid many of these problems by achieving near normal blood-sugar control before and during pregnancy. For example, infants born to mothers with diabetes have about a 10% chance of being born with a birth defect, compared with only 2% of babies born to nondiabetic mothers. These birth defects typically involve the spinal cord, the kidneys, and the heart.

This risk of birth defects can be greatly reduced, however, by achieving normal blood-sugar control before pregnancy even occurs. In fact, blood-sugar control is most important during the first 12 weeks of pregnancy because this is the time when all of the infant's major organs are formed. To be safe, you should plan on achieving an A1C level (see Glossary) within 1% of normal before you start trying to get pregnant. If successful, you will give your baby the best chance for a healthy start in life, and you will also decrease the chances of delivering a very large baby. This will improve your chances of staying healthy, too. If you're thinking about having a baby, talk with your doctor before trying to conceive so that you can work out a plan together.

162 I missed my menstrual cycle and may be pregnant. Will my diabetes medications harm my baby?

If you think you may be pregnant, it's important to see your doctor immediately so he or she can evaluate the safety of taking your oral medications. (Be sure to tell your doctor if you are planning to become pregnant.) Blood-sugar control by insulin injection during pregnancy reduces the chance of your baby gaining too much weight, having birth defects, or having high or low blood sugar. Insulin therapy is also recommended for nursing women, as the insulin does not pass into the breast milk.

Once you have delivered your baby and have stopped nursing, you should be able to discontinue insulin therapy and return to taking your oral medications. If you are using insulin prior to pregnancy, the amount needed to control your blood sugar will change during and after pregnancy. For example, you may need less insulin while breastfeeding than you were using before your pregnancy.

163 Will my diabetic kidney disease get worse if I get pregnant?

If you have kidney disease before getting pregnant, there's a 30% chance that it will worsen during pregnancy. In fact, many women with diabetes will first show signs of abnormal kidney function (releasing protein into the urine) during pregnancy. But these changes often improve after delivering the infant.

Babies born to mothers with diabetic kidney disease have a higher risk of stillbirth, respiratory distress, jaundice, and an abnormally small body size compared to babies of mothers with diabetes without kidney problems. Also, about 30% of these babies are born prematurely. You will need to have tight blood-sugar control and careful control of blood pressure before and during the pregnancy. It can be done, but know the risks before you get pregnant.

164 I have type 2 diabetes and was quite overweight when I became pregnant. Should I try to lose a few pounds for a healthier pregnancy?

No. It's true that women who are overweight during pregnancy may experience more medical problems, such as hypertension (high blood pressure) and preeclampsia (hypertension and swelling caused by pregnancy). However, pregnancy is not the time to lose weight. Cutting down on calories can cause your body to burn fat stores, resulting in ketones (a byproduct of fat metabolism), which could be harmful to your baby. Rather than dieting, try to limit your weight gain to about 15 pounds while you are pregnant. Keep your weight gain steady and vow to yourself that you'll drop the pounds after the baby is born.

165 Does getting diabetes while I'm pregnant mean that I'm more likely to get permanent diabetes later?

Yes. The fact that you get high blood sugars during pregnancy, a condition called "gestational diabetes," indicates that your pancreas cannot make enough extra insulin to cover the increased needs caused by pregnancy. This suggests that you might develop type 2 diabetes even if you never get pregnant again. Each year approximately 5% of women like you will develop diabetes if they don't make efforts to improve their lifestyles.

Women gain weight during pregnancy but do not always lose all of it after delivery. With several pregnancies, a woman may gain quite a bit of weight. Therefore, if you develop high blood sugars during pregnancy, it's very important to lose all of the weight you gained during your pregnancy. Eating healthy meals and exercising daily is the best approach to prevent permanent diabetes.

If you decide to breastfeed, do not begin a weight-loss program without medical advice. To breastfeed, you need the same number of calories that you needed during the final three months of pregnancy. When you stop breastfeeding, then you can focus on losing any extra weight you're still carrying.

PREVENTION BASICS

166 Can diabetes be prevented?

Many scientists believe that the answer is yes. Because the causes of type 1 and type 2 diabetes are different, approaches to preventing each form of diabetes are different.

Type 1 diabetes is thought to be caused by an allergic-like reaction, probably to insulin, the pancreas, or some substance in the pancreas. If this is true, then it is possible that diabetes could be prevented by giving the susceptible person small injections of insulin, much like allergy shots may prevent hay fever. This approach has been successful in animals who were bred to get diabetes. However, this approach was not successful in a National Institutes of Health clinical trial. Other approaches, such as oral insulin, are still being investigated.

Type 2 diabetes does not seem to be caused by an allergic reaction. The cause is probably related to a hereditary defect that reduces a person's sensitivity to insulin. New medications used early may prevent type 2 diabetes. Also, lifestyle changes, including exercise and weight loss, may prevent it. The Diabetes Prevention Program has recently shown that diet and exercise prevent the incidence of diabetes by about 60%, with the oral medication, metformin, preventing about 30%.

167 I have type 2 diabetes and I worry about other family members getting it. Is there any way to test them and/or prevent it?

The short answer is yes. One study was conducted involving people who were overweight and had impaired glucose tolerance (IGT), sometimes called "pre-diabetes." People with IGT have high blood-sugar levels but not high enough to be diagnosed as diabetic. About half of all people with IGT eventually develop type 2 diabetes.

Participants in the study were divided into three groups. One group received coaching in a healthy lifestyle designed to help them lose weight. The goal in this group was to be active (for most, this meant walking) 30 minutes a day, five days a week, and to lose 7% of their weight and keep it off. The other two groups took pills but made no lifestyle changes. Of these two groups, one group took a medication called "metformin" (Glucophage), and the other group took placebo pills that looked just like the metformin but had no active medication.

The results of the study were impressive. People in the group who made lifestyle changes were 58% less likely to develop diabetes during the study than the people in the placebo group. Metformin also helped prevent diabetes during this study, but it was only half as effective as lifestyle changes. So, yes, it is possible to prevent diabetes, though we don't know for how long.

168 Will losing weight decrease my risk of getting diabetes?

Yes. The Diabetes Prevention Program (DPP) shows that people with impaired glucose tolerance (IGT) who lose 10-15 pounds reduce their risk of getting type 2 diabetes by more than 50%. (Impaired glucose tolerance means your body isn't taking the glucose out of your blood as efficiently as it should.) If you are older than 60, the DPP found that losing 10-15 pounds reduced the risk of diabetes by 71%. Good news—these effects were the same for men and women and all minority groups.

In addition, one-third of the people who lost the weight and exercised at least 150 minutes per week (30 minutes five times a week) improved their blood-sugar levels from IGT to normal. So, losing weight not only helps prevent diabetes, it also helps bring elevated blood-sugar levels back to normal!

The Finnish Diabetes Prevention study had similar results. A weight loss of 11% of body weight (more than 15 pounds) was associated with more than an 80% reduced risk of getting type 2 diabetes. These results strongly suggest that the more weight you lose, the better chance you have of preventing type 2 diabetes.

169 Does exercise help prevent diabetes?

Yes. Research shows that increasing your activity level is an important lifestyle change for preventing diabetes. In the Diabetes Prevention Program (DPP), a major clinical trial, participants in the lifestyle-change group were asked to exercise at least 150 minutes a week. Most of them chose brisk walking, and others started swimming or biking. The average activity level per week was 208 minutes in the first year and 189 minutes per week at the end of the three-year study.

Another study in China showed that increasing physical activity can reduce the risk of developing diabetes by 46%. Participants in this study were asked to increase their exercise level by two units a day for those over 50 who had no problems with heart disease or arthritis (see chart on page 203). The average activity level was four units per day. The clear message is that activity alone—even without weight loss—is a powerful diabetes prevention strategy.

Activities Required for One Unit of Exercise

Intensity	Time (minutes)	Exercise
Mild	30	Slow walking, traveling, shopping, housecleaning
Moderate	20	Faster walking, going downstairs, cycling, doing heavy laundry, ballroom dancing (slow)
Strenuous	10	Slow running, climbing stairs, disco dancing for the elderly, playing volleyball or table tennis
Very strenuous	5	Jumping rope, playing basketball, swimming

The Da Qing IGT and Diabetes study. *Diabetes Care.* 1997;
20(4): 537–544.

170 If I have impaired glucose tolerance, what are my chances of getting diabetes later in life?

Impaired glucose tolerance (IGT) is a dangerous pre-diabetic condition. Reversing it with diet and exercise may prevent you from getting diabetes. IGT is a gray area between having normal blood sugar and having diabetes. If you have IGT, your pre-breakfast blood-sugar values are slightly elevated, usually above 110 mg/dl. This level is not high enough for a diagnosis of diabetes, which is blood-sugar levels above 126 mg/dl. Although you don't have diabetes, 5% of people with IGT do develop diabetes every year. This means that if you have had IGT for five years, your chances for getting diabetes increase to about 25%.

People with IGT are usually overweight, don't get much exercise, and often have relatives who have type 2 diabetes. Most doctors believe that if people with IGT improve their health by losing weight and exercising more, their chances for developing diabetes will be much lower. Also, eating a low-fat and high-fiber diet may help. It's important to get your blood-sugar level checked at least once a year, and if it is high, work on getting it into the normal range and keeping it there.

GLOSSARY

A1C test—a test that shows a person's average blood-glucose level over the previous 2-3 months, usually shown as a percentage.

ACE inhibitor—an oral medicine that lowers blood pressure. For people with diabetes, especially those who have protein (albumin) in the urine, it also helps slow down kidney damage.

albuminuria—a condition in which the urine has more than normal amounts of albumin; a frequent sign of diabetic nephropathy (kidney disease).

autoantibody—a self-recognizing antibody that targets and attacks the cells of the body, leading the body to attack itself.

blood fat—a lipid carried through the blood by a lipoprotein, usually used in reference to cholesterol and triglyceride.

blood glucose—the main sugar found in the blood and the body's main energy source; also called blood sugar.

blood-glucose level—the amount of glucose in a given amount of blood, often measured in milligrams of glucose per deciliter of blood and shown as mg/dl.

blood pressure—the force of blood exerted on the inside walls of blood vessels.

blood sugar—blood glucose.

carbohydrate—one of the three primary macronutrients found in food, primarily starches, vegetables, fruits, dairy products, and sugars.

certified diabetes educator—a health-care professional with expertise in diabetes education and who has met eligibility requirements and successfully completed a certification exam. *Abbrev.*: CDE.

cholesterol—a type of fat produced by the liver and found in the blood; it is also found in some foods; used by the body to make hormones and build cell walls.

creatinine—a waste product from protein in the diet and from the muscles of the body that is eliminated from the body by the kidneys in the form of urine; used as a marker for kidney function because as nephropathy progresses, the creatinine levels in the blood increase.

dietitian—a health-care professional who advises people about meal planning, weight control, and diabetes management. A registered dietitian (RD) has more training.

fat—1. One of the main macronutrients in food, found in butter, margarine, salad dressing, oil, nuts, meat, poultry, fish, and some dairy products.

2. Any of the different kinds of fat found in food, including monounsaturated fat, omega-e fatty acid, polyunsaturated fat, saturated fat, and trans fatty acid.

glucagon—a hormone produced by the alpha cells in the pancreas that raises blood-glucose levels. An injectable form of glucagon, available by prescription, may be used to treat severe hypoglycemia.

heart attack—an interruption in the blood supply to the heart because of narrowed or blocked blood vessels, causing muscle damage and possibly death; also called myocardial infarction.

hemoglobin—the part of a red blood cell that carries oxygen to the cells; when it joins with the glucose in the bloodstream, it is called glycosylated hemoglobin or HbA_{1c}.

hyperglycemia—a condition characterized by excessively high blood-glucose levels; signs include excessive thirst (polydipsia), excessive urination (polyuria), and excessive hunger (polyphagia).

hypoglycemia—a condition characterized by abnormally low blood-glucose levels, usually less than 70 mg/dl; signs include hunger, nervousness, shakiness, perspiration, dizziness, light-headedness, sleepiness, and confusion. If left untreated, hypoglycemia may lead to unconsciousness.

insulin—a polypeptide hormone that helps the body use glucose for energy; created by the beta cells of the pancreas. All animals (including humans) require insulin to survive.

ketone—a waste product that results from the process of the body breaking down body fat for energy, which is a situation that arises when there is a shortage of insulin. High levels can lead to diabetic ketoacidosis and coma. Also called ketone bodies.

kidney failure—a chronic condition in which the kidneys no longer work properly, resulting in the body retaining fluid and causing harmful wastes to build up inside the body; this life-threatening condition is usually treated with dialysis or a kidney transplant.

lactose—a type of sugar found in milk and milk products.

licensed practical nurse—a nurse who has received 1-2 years of training, received certification and licensing from a state authority, and works under the supervision of registered nurses and physicians. Also called licensed vocational nurse (LVN). *Abbrev.*: LPN.

lipid—a term for fat in the body, usually broken down by the body and used for energy.

lipoprotein—a protein that travels through the bloodstream with the purpose of delivering lipids to cells.

macronutrient—nutrients your body requires in large amounts, including carbohydrates, protein, and fat.

mg/dl—a measure of concentration using milligrams per deciliter.

microalbuminuria—a condition characterized by small amounts of albumin in the urine; an early sign of nephropathy; usually managed by improving blood-glucose control, reducing blood pressure, and modifying diet.

nephropathy—disease of the kidneys. Hyperglycemia and hypertension can damage the glomerulus of the kidney. When the kidneys are damaged, they can no longer remove waste and extra fluids from the bloodstream and protein leaks into the urine.

nurse practitioner—a registered nurse who has taken advanced training and received a master's degree in nursing; can perform many of the duties of a physician without supervision; may take on additional duties in diagnosis and treatment of patients.

nutritionist—a person with training in nutrition; may or may not have specialized training and qualifications (as opposed to a dietitian).

ophthalmologist—a medical doctor who diagnoses and treats all eye diseases and eye disorders; can also prescribe glasses and contact lenses.

protein—1. one of the main macronutrients in food. Foods that provide protein include meat, poultry, fish, cheese, milk, dairy products, eggs, and dried beans.
2. proteins are also used in the body for cell structure, hormones such as insulin, and other functions.

proteinuria—the presence of protein in the urine, indicating that the kidneys are not working properly.

registered dietitian—a dietitian who has had further education and training in order to earn credentials from the Commission on Accreditation for Dietetics Education, an agency of the American Dietetic Association. *Abbrev.*: RD.

retinopathy—damage to small blood vessels in the eye that can lead to vision problems; different forms include background retinopathy and proliferative retinopathy.

stroke—a serious condition caused by damage to blood vessels in the brain, which stops the flow of blood and oxygen to the brain, possibly causing brain cells to die; may cause loss of ability to speak or to move parts of the body.

triglyceride—the storage form of fat in the body.

vitamin—an organic substance that living organisms require in very small quantities for good health; normally, the organism cannot create the vitamins itself and instead must obtain it from the diet, either from foods or from dietary supplements (e.g., pills).

INDEX

meal plans. *See Meal
planning.*
protein, 61, 66, 68, 72, 81,
90, 92-94, 104
sodium intake, lowering, 95,
106
weight reduction, 108-114,
120
Doctor visits,
checklist for, 32
frequency of, 31, 45

E

Erectile dysfunction, 169
Exercise,
arthritis and, 128, 202
athletic shoes, 182
benefits, 122, 159, 202, 204
blood-sugar testing before,
125-126
to decrease blood pressure,
98
to IGT, reversing, 191
stopping medications and,
142
Eye problems, 139, 153 169,
185
blindness, 25, 36, 185
cataracts, 123, 185
exams and, 32, 45
exercise and, 123
floaters, 185
macular edema, 185
retinopathy, 123, 185

F

Fainting spells, 168
Fats
Monounsaturated, 101-102
Omega-3, 84
Polyunsaturated, 101-102
Saturated, 71, 83, 93-94,
98, 101, 104
Trans, 83
Fat replacers, 81-82
Fiber, dietary, 53, 88-90, 93,
104
Fingernails, fungal infections
of, 187
Fish oil, 84, 154
Floaters, 183
Food and Drug Administration,
67, 153, 191
Food labels, 67, 79
Foot care, 165
athlete's foot, 187
daily examination, 173
numbness, 177
peripheral neuropathy, 166,
168, 178
painful neuropathy, 176
shoes, 124, 175, 182
Frank, Johann Peter, 21
Fructose, 70, 77, 96
Fungal infections, 187

G

Glipizide, 146
Glucophage, 145, 167
Glyburide, 138, 141, 146